Midwifery Care for Pregnant Women Who Live with Obesity

This practical guide equips midwives with the skills and knowledge necessary to support pregnant women living with obesity, from communicating meaningfully about weight through to providing evidence-based information about optimising health and making changes.

Beginning with an overview of what living with obesity means for women, this book supports midwives to develop consultation skills and structure their encounters with women for maximum effect. It presents up-to-date, evidence-based information about the impact of obesity on pregnant women and their unborn babies from conception to birth and beyond. Chapters on changing health behaviours, nutrition and physical activity explore how to mitigate these risks and optimise health.

Including reflective questions and case studies, this book is designed for practising and student midwives looking to develop their personalised care and communication skills.

Yvonne M. Greig has been practicing as a midwife since 1991. Since 2000, she has combined academic and clinical practice and has enjoyed practicing in varied roles. In 2011, she became the lead midwife for the Metabolic Antenatal Clinic at the University of Edinburgh/NHS Lothian where care was provided for women who lived with raised body mass index. This clinic conducted many research studies that explored the impact of living with obesity. It was here that Yvonne became interested in the professional practice surrounding the topic and became curious as to why many women had not been told of the risks that living with obesity brought. This curiosity led to doctoral work and has culminated in the publication of this book. Along the way, Yvonne has also worked in Kenya as part of the Liverpool School of Tropical Medicine, delivering education to healthcare professionals with respect to providing maternity care. She has also liaised with colleagues in Greece and supported the development of a midwifery degree course there and has supported the British University of Egypt with modules concerned with family care and health. Currently, Yvonne is a midwifery researcher and lecturer at Edinburgh Napier University.

Midwifery Care for Pregnant Women Who Live with Obesity

A Guide to Explaining the Risks and Providing Practical Advice

Yvonne M. Greig

Routledge
Taylor & Francis Group
LONDON AND NEW YORK

First published 2024
by Routledge
4 Park Square, Milton Park, Abingdon, Oxon OX14 4RN

and by Routledge
605 Third Avenue, New York, NY 10158

Routledge is an imprint of the Taylor & Francis Group, an informa business

British Library Cataloguing-in-Publication Data
A catalogue record for this book is available from the British Library

Library of Congress Cataloging-in-Publication Data
Names: Greig, Yvonne M., author.
Title: Midwifery care for pregnant women who live with obesity : a guide to explaining the risks and providing practical advice / Yvonne M. Greig.
Description: Abingdon, Oxon ; New York, NY : Routledge, 2024. |
Includes bibliographical references and index. Identifiers: LCCN 2023047835 (print) |
LCCN 2023047836 (ebook) |
ISBN 9781032365138 (hbk) | ISBN 9781032365114 (pbk) |
ISBN 9781003332398 (ebk)
Subjects: LCSH: Pregnant women--Weight gain. | Pregnancy--Nutritional aspects. | Prenatal care. | Overweight women. | Obesity in women.
Classification: LCC RG559 .G74 2024 (print) | LCC RG559 (ebook) |
DDC 618.2/42--dc23/eng/20231205
LC record available at https://lccn.loc.gov/2023047835
LC ebook record available at https://lccn.loc.gov/2023047836

ISBN: 978-1-032-36513-8 (hbk)
ISBN: 978-1-032-36511-4 (pbk)
ISBN: 978-1-003-33239-8 (ebk)

DOI: 10.4324/9781003332398

Typeset in Sabon
by SPi Technologies India Pvt Ltd (Straive)

This book is dedicated to the late Professor Fiona Denison, University of Edinburgh, who was a friend, colleague and supporter.

Contents

Tables

Boxes

Introduction

Aim of the Book

Obesity is a serious public health concern, but despite this understanding, rates of obesity are still high, although they do now appear to be stabilising. This book is not intended to be a prescriptive manual providing professionals with absolute scripts about what midwives should or should not say to women and their families who might live a with raised weight. Rather, it is intended to strengthen one's underpinning knowledge about the various issues pertaining to living with obesity during pregnancy and how to engage in meaningful conversations about how to mitigate the risks of living with an unhealthy weight. It is hoped that utilising this book will strengthen knowledge and practice not only about the topic of obesity itself and its potential risks to women and children but also with respect to constructing meaningful consultation episodes.

The Scope and Severity of Obesity

Obesity has been described by the World Health Organization (WHO) (2021) as a major risk for non-communicable disease and carries significant health risks such as cardiovascular disease, osteoarthritis, cancers and type II diabetes, to name a few. Although obesity rates in the UK are now levelling (Baker 2023), they have risen over the last five decades, meaning that populations continue to be burdened by obesity-related disease. In 2016, it was estimated that 39% of adults were overweight and that 13% were obese (WHO 2021). In England, the levels of obesity between those 16 to 44 years of age range from 37% to 64% (for men and women) (Baker 2023), and similar levels are seen across the other three UK nations. These figures suggest that a significant proportion of childbearing women will be living with obesity. Furthermore, the WHO estimated that more than 340 million children and young people 5 to 19 years of age were either overweight or obese (WHO 2021). It is likely that some of these overweight or obese young people will go on to become overweight or obese parents themselves, meaning that the cycle of obesity and related ill health is likely to continue.

The leading cause of obesity is an energy imbalance (WHO 2021). That is, the energy that is taken in is more than the energy expended. Whilst it is recognised that there are some genetic conditions that increase the risk of an individual's becoming obese, the main causes are environmental, such as the easy availability of obesogenic foods in the developed world and a trend towards more sedentary lifestyles and changes to family eating patterns (Lean & Combet 2017). Although obesity is considered to be a preventable condition, Lim et al. (2020) suggest that, once developed, it is difficult to reverse.

DOI: 10.4324/9781003332398-1

Living with obesity brings risks to women during pregnancy, labour and birth, such as hypertension, gestational diabetes, miscarriage, pre-term labour and an increased need for Caesarean section (C/S) (Denison et al. 2009; Arrowsmith & Quenby 2011; Denison & Chiswick 2011; Knight 2019). Unborn babies too are at risk of developing foetal anomalies, the most common of which are cardiac defects and cleft lip and palate. Macrosomia is also a risk for these babies, which in turn increases the risks of birth injury occurring and of the need for admission to the neonatal unit (Drake & Reynolds 2010; Stirrat & Reynolds 2014). Furthermore, empirical evidence suggests that children who are born to women who live with a body mass index (BMI) of at least 30 kg/m^2 are at increased risk of experiencing adult obesity and ongoing poor health throughout the lifelong continuum (Catalano et al. 2009; Stirrat & Reynolds 2014). It is believed that this is as a result of the phenomenon known as 'early life programming', in which the foetus adapts to a sup-optimal environment in order to survive (Lean & Combet 2017). This epigenetic adaptation is thought to play a role in susceptibility to disease for the offspring throughout the lifelong continuum because of changes to both DNA and micro-RNA (Şanlı & Kabaran 2019). These findings suggest that if this public health problem is not addressed, future generations will continue to be at risk of sub-optimal health as a result of their parents' obesity. This, in turn, means that the burden of disease for individuals and populations alike will continue to challenge governments as they plan healthcare provision in the face of ongoing spiralling costs.

In the UK, we live in a society where there is easy access to affordable, obesogenic foods and where foods high in sugar and fats are being strategically placed in supermarkets, thus influencing people to perhaps make sub-optimal dietary choices (Obesity Health Alliance 2018). In addition, there is little focus upon the strategic placement of healthy foods (in the UK), meaning that this may be influencing and compounding the sub-optimal choices that some individuals make. This undoubtedly will include some pregnant women who are unknowingly putting themselves at greater risk of pregnancy complications whilst continuing to set the unborn baby on a sub-optimal lifelong continuum with respect to both childhood and adult health (Lean & Combet 2017).

Current Midwifery Practice

Most pregnant women in the UK will see a midwife throughout their pregnancy for antenatal appointments. According to the Independent Maternity Review (2022), every antenatal appointment should be considered an opportunity to undertake a risk assessment to promote the mother and baby's safety, and healthcare professionals (HCPs) need to recognise that risk is not static but dynamic and can change over time (Knight et al. 2019). If the midwife identifies risk factors for the mother and/or baby, then he/she has a professional responsibility to discuss them and, depending on severity, refer the woman to specialist services for care planning (Nursing and Midwifery Council [NMC] 2019). However, prior to making a referral, the midwife must explain his/her actions, and in the context of identifying an obese woman, this means raising and discussing the topics of weight management, diet and physical activity as well as seeking consent to make the referral.

If they are to engage in meaningful conversations with women who live with obesity, midwives need to be in possession of appropriate knowledge regarding the complex issues that surround the condition in order to give appropriate advice with respect to protecting current health and promoting future health for both mother and child. However, there remains a challenge for professionals because national guidance documents (Denison et al. 2019) suggest that women *'should'* be informed of the incumbent risks of living with obesity and offered additional foetal and maternal monitoring, but these documents do not inform professionals *how* to raise the apparently sensitive issues that surround being overweight or obese.

Despite the duty of care that midwives have to promote safety for mother and baby, tensions appear to exist, and midwives are reluctant to raise the topic for fear of damaging the midwife–woman relationship, a force that is being promoted as positive in a woman's life (Scottish Government 2017; NHS England 2017). Reasons found for evading this topic are lack of knowledge, lack of confidence, and fear of damaging the midwife–woman relationship (Lutsiv et al. 2012; Macleod et al. 2013; Singleton & Furber 2014; Arrish et al. 2016; McParlin et al. 2017).

The Role of the Professional

Midwives and other HCPs alone cannot alter the rising obesity rates which challenge both individual and public health. The problems that led to an increase in obesity rates are multi-factorial, economic and social (Lean & Combet 2017; WHO 2021). However, professionals can be part of the solution by developing appropriate consultation skills that will facilitate meaningful conversations about living with obesity, which include accurate information about how to mitigate the potential complications that living with an unhealthy weight can cause. Indeed, midwives have a professional responsibility to share evidence-based information with the families in their care, as can be seen from the following quote from the NMC of the UK:

> demonstrate the ability to share information on public health, health promotion and health protection with women, enabling them to make evidence-informed decisions, and providing support for access to resources and services
>
> (NMC 2019, p. 19)

If midwives are to meet the above-mentioned professional standard (NMC 2019), they will also need to be in possession of appropriate knowledge and understanding about the implications of living with obesity and how making positive lifestyle choices can improve health.

Identifying the Obese Individual

In order to discuss the implications of living with obesity with women, one first has to identify whether someone meets the criteria to be overweight or obese. The BMI, a simple and cost-effective calculation, is an individual's weight (kg) divided by their height in metres squared (m^2). This calculation was developed during the 1830s by the Belgian mathematician Adolphe Quetelet in an attempt to identify the 'ideal' weight' (Romero-Corral et al. 2008). Since its development, this calculation has been adopted in healthcare settings as a diagnostic rather than a screening tool. Subsequently, the majority of weight-related research pertaining to the implications of living with obesity (for both non-pregnant and pregnant populations) is based on the BMI measurement. It is, however, a blunt instrument and does not distinguish between lean or fat mass, genders or ethnicities, meaning that some individuals may be labelled as being overweight or obese when they instead have high muscularity.

Understanding that the BMI calculation is not a perfect gauge of an individual's body mass is important for clinical practice, particularly when faced with a 'borderline' BMI of 30–35 kg/m^2, for example. In such cases, it is vital that the woman's personal context be explored in some detail, taking into account her lifestyle, diet and physical activity. When a BMI is raised (35 kg/m^2 and over), it may be easier to visually assess someone's level of adiposity; however, exploring the woman's personal context is still necessary and will go some way to ensuring that appropriate and person-centred advice is provided.

Making use of anthropometric measurements (skinfold thickness and waist, leg and arm circumferences) may go some way to overcoming the challenges associated with BMI measurement. However, this is dependent upon using the correctly calibrated equipment and ensuring that staff are well educated with the appropriate skills in obtaining accurate body measurements and understand the calculations necessary to discern whether an individual is 'obese' or not. Furthermore, as pregnancy progresses, the waist circumference will be inaccurate because the uterus is expanding into the abdomen. It may also be necessary for health authorities to purchase expensive scales and other equipment that calculate body composition. This throws up challenges of payment and ownership, especially in shared clinical spaces, and anxieties about equipment being inappropriately used or lost. For reasons mentioned above, the BMI measurement will be referred to in this book. However, it will be wise to be cognisant of the potential shortcomings of this calculation and keep in mind that care provision must be person-centred and take into account the individual's personal context.

The Language of Weight and Fat Stigma

'Fat stigma' has gathered some attention in recent years and is associated with the negative stereotypes, characteristics and associations associated with being fat (Pause 2017), meaning that often people who live with higher weights are labelled as being lazy or of lower intelligence and, as a result, may be provided with inferior healthcare services (Christenson et al. 2018). Furthermore, 'fat stigma' has been found to increase the risk of binge eating, mental health disorders and the rejection of healthcare advice (Williams & Annandale 2019). Sensitivity and compassion therefore are required values of the professional when introducing personal conversations about living with obesity, and it is these personalised conversations that Saw et al. (2021) concluded may result in women's positively receiving the advice on offer.

Brown and Flint (2021) assert that how the topic is raised and the language within conversations about living with obesity can either engage and motivate the individual or have the opposite effect. Brown and Flint (2021) found that terms most acceptable to individuals who lived with obesity were 'weight', 'unhealthy weight' and 'overweight' and appeared to evoke less negative emotions than the words 'obese', 'fat' and 'chubby'. These findings are noteworthy and in light of this evidence, it is recommended that the terms 'weight', 'overweight' and 'unhealthy weight' be used when providing advice to women.

Overview of Book

Chapter 1 discusses some of the theory that surrounds 'consultation' and the models currently used in medical practice. It gives some guidance about how these consultation models may be appropriately adapted for use in midwifery practice and discusses the 'flipped consultation'.

Chapters 2 and 3 explore and discuss the risks (to both mother and baby) associated with living with obesity during pregnancy, labour and birth and ongoing risks to the child throughout the lifelong continuum. There is acknowledgement of recent findings with respect to maternal diet in early pregnancy and 'programming' that may predispose the unborn child to obesity. Despite these alarming findings, it is now understood that making positive lifestyle choices with respect to diet and physical activity can reduce risk and improve pregnancy outcomes. Chapters 4 and 5 discusses these issues in some detail.

Chapter 4 provides an overview of nutrition, the components of diet that are required to maintain good health and the foods that these nutrients are found in. It discusses the optimum weight gain for pregnant women. This chapter offers advice to midwives about the dietary advice they should be providing for all women but particularly those who live with an unhealthy weight.

Chapter 5 discusses what benefits of engaging in physical activity and the current UK recommendations for physical activity for women during pregnancy. There is some discussion about how midwives can encourage women to engage in physical activity. Although exercise is recommended for all, some women during pregnancy may develop a condition or live with chronic conditions that preclude them from exercising. These conditions are also discussed.

Chapter 6 provides an overview of some of the key papers that have informed us about the risks of living with obesity and why this topic is one that we should not shy away from. It should be noted that this is not a literature review but a summary of key studies that have been conducted about the risks of living with obesity.

Chapter 7 discusses how pre-conceptual care might be effective in informing and supporting obese pregnant women to optimise their general health and their weight prior to conception. Discussion about the challenges of providing such a service is included. The second part of the chapter briefly discusses eating disorders and advises midwives that women who live with raised BMI may be at risk of eating disorders and therefore malnourishment. This is not a comprehensive discussion on the topic; that is beyond the scope of this book. However, it is anticipated that this will draw the topic to the midwives' attention and alert them that these conditions exist and that some women will require support.

References

Arrish, J., Yeatman, H., & Williamson, M. (2016). Australian midwives and provision of nutrition education during pregnancy: A cross sectional survey of nutrition knowledge, attitudes and confidence. *Women and Birth*, *29*, 455–464. https://doi.org/10.1016/j.wombi.2016.03.001

Arrowsmith, W. S., & Quenby, S. (2011). Maternal obesity and labour complications following induction of labour in prolonged pregnancy. *BJOG: An International Journal of Obstetrics and Gynaecology*, *118*(5), 578–588. https://doi.org/10.1111/j.1471-0528.2010.02889.x

Baker, C. (2023). Obesity statistics. House of Commons Library. https://researchbriefings.files.parliament.uk/documents/SN03336/SN03336.pdf

Brown, A., & Flint, S. W. (2021). *Preferences and emotional response to weight-related terminology used by healthcare professionals to describe body weight in people living with overweight and obesity*. Wiley. https://doi.org/10.1111/cob.12470

Catalano, P., Presley, L., Minium, J., & Haugal-De-Mouzon, S. (June, 2009). Fetuses of obese mothers develop insulin resistance in utero. *Diabetes Care* [Online], *32*(6), 1076–1080. Retrieved from January 15, 2016.

Christenson, A., Johansson, E., Reynisdottir, S., Torgerson, J., & Hemmingsson, E. (2018). Shame and avoidance as barriers in midwives' communication about body weight with pregnant women: A qualitative interview study. *Midwifery*, *63*, 1–7. https://doi.org/10.1016/j.midw.2018.04.020

Denison, A. N. R., Keag, O., Hor, K., Reynolds, R. M., Milne, A., & Diamond, A. (2019). Care of women with obesity in pregnancy: Green-top guideline no. 72. *BJOG: An International Journal of Obstetrics and Gynaecology*, *126*(3), e62–e106. https://doi.org/10.1111/1471-0528.15386

Denison, F., Norrie, G., Graham, B., Lynch, J., Harper, N., & Reynolds, R. (2009). Increased maternal BMI is associated with an increased risk of minor complications during pregnancy with consequent cost implications. *BJOG: An International Journal of Obstetrics and Gynaecology*, *116*(11), 1467–1472. https://doi.org/10.1111/j.1471-0528.2009.02222.x

Denison, F. C., & Chiswick, C. (2011). Improving pregnancy outcome in obese women. *The Proceedings of the Nutrition Society*, *70*(4), 457–464. https://doi.org/10.1017/S0029665111001637

Drake, A. J., & Reynolds, R. M. (2010). Impact of maternal obesity on offspring obesity and cardiometabolic disease risk. *Reproduction* (Cambridge, England), *140*(3), 387–398. https://doi.org/10.1530/rep-10-0077

Independent Maternity Review. (2022). Ockenden report – Final: Findings, conclusions, and essential actions from the independent review of maternity services at the Shrewsbury and Telford Hospital NHS Trust (HC 1219). Crown.

Knight, M. (2019). MBRRACE-UK update: Key messages from the UK and Ireland confidential enquiries into maternal death and morbidity 2018. *The Obstetrician & Gynaecologist*, *21*(1), 69–71. https://doi.org/10.1111/tog.12548

Lean, M. E. J., & Combet, E. (2017). *Barasi's human nutrition. A health perspective* (3rd ed.). CRC Press. https://doi.org/10.1201/9781315380728

Lim, H. J., Xue, H., & Wang, Y. (2020). Global trends in obesity. In H. Meiselman (Eds.), *Handbook of eating and drinking. Springer*. https://doi.org/10.1007/978-3-030-14504-0_157

Lutsiv, O., Bracken, K., Pullenayegum, E., Sword, W., Taylor, V. H., & McDonald, S. D. (2012). Little congruence between health care provider and patient perceptions of counselling on gestational weight gain. *Journal of Obstetrics and Gynaecology*, *34*(6), 518–524. https://doi.org/10.1016/S1701-2163(16)35267-7

MacLeod, M., Gregor, A., Barnett, C., Magee, E., Thompson, J., & Anderson, A. S. (2013). Provision of weight management advice for obese women during pregnancy: A survey of current practice and midwives' views on future approaches. *Maternal & Child Nutrition*, *9*(4), 467–472. https://doi.org/10.1111/j.1740-8709.2011.00396.x

McParlin, C., Bell, R., Robson, S. C., Muirhead, C. R., & Araujo-Soares, V. (2017). What helps or hinders midwives to implement physical activity guidelines for obese pregnant women? A questionnaire survey using the Theoretical Domains Framework. *Midwifery*, *49*, 110–116. https://doi.org/10.1016/j.midw.2016.09.015

NHS England (2017). Better Births: Improving maternity services in England. Retrieved 4th December 2023, from https://www.england.nhs.uk/publication/better-births-improving-outcomes-of-maternity-services-in-england-a-five-year-forward-view-for-maternity-care/

Nursing and Midwifery Council. (2019). Standards of proficiency for midwives [online]. Retrieved November 28, 2019, from https://www.nmc.org.uk/standards/midwifery/education

Obesity Health Alliance. (2018). *Out of Place*. Accessed December 2nd, from, https://obesityhealthalliance.org.uk/wp-content/uploads/2018/11/Out-of-Place-Obesity-Health-Alliance-2.pdf

Pause, C. (2017). Borderline: The ethics of fat stigma in public health. *Journal of Law, Medicine and Ethics*, *45*, 510–517. https://doi.org/10.1177/1073110517750585

Romero-Corral, A., Somers, V. K., Sierra-Johnson, J., Thomas, R. J., Collazo-Clavell, M. L., Korinek, J., Allison, T. G., Batsis, J. A., Sert-Kuniyoshi, F. H., & Lopez-Jimenez, F. (2008). Accuracy of body mass index in diagnosing obesity in the adult general population. *International Journal of Obesity*, *32*(6), 959–966. https://doi.org/10.1038/ijo.2008.11

Şanlı, E., & Kabaran, S. (2019). Maternal obesity, maternal overnutrition and fetal programming: Effects of epigenetic mechanisms on the development of metabolic disorders. *Current Genomics*, *20*(6), 419–427. https://doi.org/10.2174/1389202920666191030092225

Saw, L., Aung, W., & Sweet, L. (2021). What the experiences of women with obesity receiving antenatal maternity care? A scoping review of qualitative evidence. *Women and Birth*, *34*, 435–446. https://doi.org/10.1016/j.wombi.2020.09.014

Singleton, G., & Furber, C. (2014). The experiences of midwives when caring for obese women in labour, a qualitative study. *Midwifery*, *30*(1), 103–111.

Stirrat, L. I., & Reynolds, R. M. (2014). Effects of maternal obesity on early and long-term outcomes for offspring. *Research and Reports in Neonatology*, *4*, 43–53. https://doi.org/10.1016/j.midw.2013.02.008

The Best Start: A 5 year forward plan for maternity and neonatal care in Scotland. (2017). Scottish Government. Retrieved from https://www.gov.scot/publications/best-start-five-year-forward-plan-maternity-neonatal-care-scotland

Williams, & Annandale, E. (2019). Weight bias internalization as an embodied process: Understanding how obesity stigma gets under the skin. *Frontiers in Psychology*, *10*, 953–953. https://doi.org/10.3389/fpsyg.2019.00953

World Health Organisation. (2021). *Overweight and Obesity*. Retrieved from https://www.who.int/news-room/fact-sheets/detail/obesity-and-overweight

1 Consultation Models

Introduction

This chapter explores the differences between communication and consultation. It explores what consultation models are and focuses on two particular models that may be helpful in underpinning conversations in a maternity care context. It goes on to analyse the various components of a consultation episode and how they might be handled in a structured framework. Some discussion is given with respect to the professional expectations of midwives and why the topic of obesity needs to be addressed at an early point in pregnancy. Examples of potential dialogue are provided as sample statements about how to inform a woman that she is living with an unhealthy weight.

Communication and Consultation

We navigate our way through life by 'communicating' or sharing our stories or 'narratives' with the people we meet in various contexts every day: social, personal and professional. These conversations take place with both the people we know and those we meet by chance. The way we communicate with our close friends and family members, however, is likely to differ from the way we speak to professionals such as a family solicitor or medical practitioner. In other words, we change our communication style depending upon the context. It is incumbent that we, as healthcare professionals, become skilled and reflective practitioners with respect to how we communicate and consult with women, pregnant people and their families, so that we effectively engage in 'uncomfortable conversations' such as the topic of obesity.

At its most simple, communication is the passing of messages from one individual to another by using speech[1] (Jomeen 2017). Communicating in a professional healthcare context, however, can be challenging and needs to be formal and precise, particularly if we are introducing a sensitive or uncomfortable topic to the dialogue. However, in the context of a maternity care consultation, we also need to hear the woman's voice so that after discussion, care planning is shared and the woman or pregnant person feels involved in clinical decision-making. During maternity care encounters, we act as consultants: experts who can provide specific advice with respect to a particular topic or topics (Collins English Dictionary). Witt and Jorgensen (2016) further define the consultation episode as a meeting between two people: one seeking help (the patient, woman or pregnant person) and the other the provider of that help (the doctor or

DOI: 10.4324/9781003332398-2

healthcare professional). A midwifery consultation, however, differs from this; here is one possible definition:

> A meeting between the midwife and the woman (and family) where open, frank and effective conversations take place aimed at exploring all aspects of the woman's health and life to ensure that accurate information about her is received and accurate, evidence-based health information is provided to her. The aim is to support a healthy pregnancy journey that will result in the woman having a safe and positive pregnancy and giving birth to a healthy baby.

Global literature has identified that midwives find discussing obesity and its incumbent risks difficult and are reluctant to raise the topic for fear of causing offence (Heslehurst et al. 2013; Knight-Agarwal et al. 2014; McParlin et al. 2017) and damaging the midwife–woman relationship, a relationship that is considered a positive force in a woman's life (NHS England 2017; Scottish Government 2017).

Furthermore, Greig et al. (2021) found that dialogue during antenatal appointments was guided by institutional questionnaires rather than being person-centred and focused on the woman's individual needs. They concluded that practicing in this way risked not viewing the woman as an individual and conflated her needs to a routinised list of problems and questions. This practice is diametrically opposed to the woman-centred approach that should now be adopted for future maternity care (NHS England 2017; Nursing and Midwifery Council [NMC] 2019; Scottish Government 2017). One also needs to consider that the NMC (2019) expects midwives to use evidence-based communication skills when sharing information with women and their families.

In addition to these professional expectations, the Montgomery ruling, a supreme court ruling, asserted that prior to accepting care all (healthcare) service users (in the UK) should be given full and detailed information with respect to any identified risk factors in order to make an informed choice based upon all of the facts and risk factors (Chan et al. 2017). Therefore, no matter how uncomfortable it may be, we need to strengthen our skills in order to have the ability to competently inform pregnant women who live with an unhealthy weight about the potential risks they face because there is little doubt that living with an unhealthy weight during pregnancy carries risks for mothers and babies.

Midwives now have a professional obligation to act as public health agents and provide relevant and evidence-based information that may improve population health NMC (2019). Therefore, discussing weight and weight management has to be on the agenda so that women are aware of how to set their child on a healthy lifetime trajectory with respect to diet and physical activity.

In the context of midwifery practice, there is now a clear understanding that we must work in partnership with women and their families to ensure that they are well informed and involved in any care decisions that are made during their maternity journey (NHS England 2017; Scottish Government 2017; NMC 2019). However, Witt and Jorgensen (2016) assert that the consultation episode is asymmetrical because one party (the professional) has more knowledge about a particular topic than the other (the patient). This asymmetry, it is suggested, causes a power imbalance (Witt & Jorgensen 2016; Launer 2018), but according to Launer (2018), by being a self-aware professional, one can manage this imbalance and facilitate the patient's voice to be heard. This is important in maternity care settings where there is an expectation that a meaningful relationship will be built with the woman who will be a partner in her own care and that her voice will be heard (NHS England 2017; The Scottish Government 2017).

Consultation Episodes

The consultation episode in healthcare has attracted interest in medical schools and in the medical profession (Silverman et al. 2013; Meitter & Karnieli-Miller 2021; Witt & Jorgensen 2016), and educators and assessors now understand that to raise some topics is difficult and can significantly and negatively impact upon the professional, the relationship with the patient and the patient himself (or pregnant woman or person) (Meitter & Karnieli-Miller 2021). As a result, 'consultation models' have been developed; these frameworks provide a structure on which to build dialogue about various topics.

In the 21st century, it is not clear what education midwives have been exposed to with respect to constructing systematic, evidence-based consultation episodes. Greig et al. (2021) found that antenatal appointments were approached in a conversational manner and that the prescriptive institutional questionnaires were used to guide dialogue. Whilst this approach may ensure that all questions pertaining to personal, medical, social and obstetric history are answered using a 'tick box' formula, it does not allow for the critical exploration of an individual's personal context.

Consultation is a complex process that combines human interaction, information sharing and the planning of care (Denness 2013). The reason that pregnant women and people generally access healthcare is not to address an illness or healthcare concern but rather to have their (usually normal) pregnancies monitored. This essentially 'flips' the consultation, with the professional being the one to identify and raise any health risk issues such as obesity, which hitherto may not have been considered troublesome by the woman.

At their core, a consultation episode is aimed at elucidating the reason for accessing healthcare, finding a diagnosis or probable diagnosis and then developing an action plan in partnership with the patient. Essentially, consultation episodes consist of three phases: a 'beginning' where introductions are made, a 'middle' where information is exchanged, and the closing phase where a diagnosis and plan of action are agreed upon (Denness 2013). Medical consultation models have been defined as having 'habits', either 5 or 6, all of which include making introductions, identifying the issue, 'listening' for additional concerns, making a diagnosis, making a plan and then closing the session. A summary of some of these frameworks can be seen in Table 1.1.

The Midwifery or 'Flipped' Consultation

Pregnancy is not generally considered an illness where medical input is required. However, women are advised to seek healthcare advice, and in the UK, it is usually the midwife who is the first professional point of contact. The first antenatal appointment or 'booking' appointment is lengthy, and a full personal, social, medical and obstetric history is sought in addition to a physical examination which will include the measurement of body mass index (BMI) (Denison et al. 2018). The aim of the appointment is to elucidate information about the woman and her family, and it is during the information exchange phase of the consultation episode that the healthcare professional is likely to identify areas of the woman's life and lifestyles that may complicate the pregnancy. Unlike in a traditional medical consultation, it is the midwife who needs to raise and maintain dialogue about sensitive issues; therefore, working within an evidence-based framework may facilitate and strengthen midwifery practice.

The Calgary-Cambridge model of consultation (Silverman et al. 2013) is a 'Five Habits' model that is patient-centred and offers a flexible but structured approach to

Table 1.1 Summary of consultation models

Name of author	*Consultation phases*
Byrne-Long (2000, as cited in Dennes 2013)	1. Rapport is formed with the patient. 2. The doctor attempts to identify the reason for attendance. 3. An examination is performed. 4. Consideration is given to the problem with or without patient involvement. 5. A care plan is made with or without the patient's involvement. 6. The doctor ends the consultation.
Pendleton (1984 as cited in Dennes 2013)	1. Reasons for attending are clarified. 2. Additional problems (if any) are identified. 3. A management plan is decided upon. 4. Working in partnership with the patient to agree on a shared understanding of the problems 5. The patient is involved in the management plan.
Neighbour (2005)	1. The doctor connects with the patient. 2. The doctor clarifies the problem and summarises it to the patient. 3. Both doctor and patient formulate a plan together with the patient making informed decisions about how to progress their care. 4. A contingency plan or 'safety netting' is set, ensuring that the patient knows where to seek additional help and care. 5. 'House keeping' – a term used to ensure that the professional acknowledges his/her own emotions about the consultation prior to the next appointment
Calgary-Cambridge (2008 as cited in Dennes 2013)	1. Initiation of the session – establishing rapport and setting the agenda for the appointment 2. Gathering information – The problem is explored using both open and closed questions and observing body language and linguistical nuances. 3. Physical examination 4. Provision of information 'in chunks' rather than one narrative at the end 5. Session is closed by summarising the events and agreeing on a clear plan. ***In addition, this model advocates for building a rapport and structure as the consultation develops.***

Table adapted from Dennes (2013).

listening, history taking and information giving, whilst, as already mentioned, developing a supportive rapport with individuals; this aligns to the philosophy of midwives building a supportive relationship with women (NHS England 2017; Scottish Government 2017). Silverman et al. (2013) also assert that in order for this model to be effective, individuals (women and pregnant people) must be given space and time to voice their concerns. Thus, active listening is also an important component of the consultation episode and is alluded to in the Calgary-Cambridge model (Silverman et al., 2013). The five phases of this model are initiating the session, information gathering, the physical examination, explanation and planning, and closing the session (Silverman et al. 2013). In a midwifery context, however, one might replace the *information gathering* phase with *information exchange* or *information sharing*; the professional can then capitalise on the opportunity to discuss what may be difficult or sensitive issues. Prior to entering this phase of the encounter, however, the professional should inform the woman about what is to come and gain her consent prior to embarking on the topic in question (in this case, living with obesity).

Breaking Bad News

Whilst it may seem that to inform someone that their increased weight may cause health issues during pregnancy is not as serious as informing them that they have acquired a life-limiting illness, a similar emotional response may be elicited when discussing such news. Being prepared for this and understanding how to deal with it may support practice and facilitate meaningful dialogue.

Meitter and Karnieli-Miller (2021) provide comprehensive tips for breaking bad news in an oncology context (although bad news can come in many guises). These tips include preparation of self, consideration of the setting, warning the patient about what is to come, validating emotional responses, discussing treatment options, providing ongoing contingency, documenting the session and, crucially, investing in critical reflection at the end of the session.

Although the two models (Meitter and Karnieli-Miller 2021; Silverman et al., 2013) differ, similarities can be drawn between them. In both, there is a focus upon listening to the individual and developing a collaborative relationship to bring about optimal outcomes. Therefore, developing a 'hybrid' of the two models may be useful for constructing antenatal consultation episodes.

Suggested Structure of an Antenatal Appointment

The following model has been developed as a loose guide for practitioners with respect to structuring a conversation pertaining to a sensitive topic. It is not a definitive 'recipe' but rather a list of tips that some may find useful. It must also be borne in mind that whilst the focus here is on the Calgary-Cambridge model (Silverman et al. 2013) and Meitter and Karnieli-Miller's (2021) tips for breaking bad news, other consultation models may suit different personalities and different contexts (Denness 2013); therefore, it may be useful to broaden one's knowledge about the other models available.

Prior to the Session

- Prepare oneself. This doesn't pertain to just preparing any relevant documentation, although that is important; rather, it is about emotionally preparing for the conversations that may develop. There is a higher chance that by taking a few minutes to do this, you will be 'present' and employ active listening during the encounter itself (Meitter & Karnieli-Miller 2021).
- Glean as much information as possible prior to the encounter. This may not be possible if the woman is attending for antenatal care for the first time, but it is worth doing and ultimately will save time during the appointment itself.

Initiating the Session

- Meitter and Karnieli-Miller (2021) suggest that when breaking bad news the professional should be aware of the setting, providing a quiet space for people. In the context of maternity care, this isn't always possible, although some appointments may take place in the woman's own home. However, even in a busy clinical area, it is important to ensure that there is adequate seating for all, that there will be no interruptions and that there are tissues at hand (in the anticipation of a negative emotional response).
- Welcome the woman and her family members and ensure their comfort. Bharj and Daniels (2017) suggest that maintaining a friendly and non-judgemental demeanour is

important in order to make women feel at ease during any antenatal appointment but especially the first one, where the parties may not have met previously.

- Introducing oneself. This may seem obvious, but Granger (2014), in her interactions with healthcare professionals, felt dehumanised when professionals did not introduce themselves by name.
- Clarifying one's role: this may be less necessary in midwifery contexts. After all, the woman has accessed maternity care, and in UK contexts, the role of the midwife is well understood. Nevertheless, it is important to explain what aspects of her care one will be involved in, particularly if practicing as part of a team or covering for sickness or leave. The woman has a right to understand where individual practitioners will fit in to her care and if they will see the same midwife at every appointment, including during labour and birth and in the postnatal period.
- Ensure that one is meeting the correct person and address them and their family members by their preferred name(s).
- Be engaged and present; ensure that any computers are switched off or turned away initially so that the individual can have confidence that they will be listened to.
- Prepare the woman and her family about what is to come. Ask if she is aware of what will be discussed and inform her about the sometimes lengthy nature of the appointment (the booking appointment) and what information will be exchanged. At this early point, inform her (and family members) that you may raise topics she hadn't expected and that some of them may benefit from a further exploration. For example:

> During your appointment, some issues may be identified that may, in the future, cause complications during your pregnancy; if so, I'd like to discuss these in more detail with you. Some of these things are smoking, your weight and your diet. Were you aware of that?

Following such a statement, remain silent and allow the woman (or family members) the space and time to process the information and then to speak and give their opinions.

Although it may be beneficial not to use the institutional questionnaires to guide dialogue, they are necessary and have an important role to ensure that critical information is gathered in order to provide safe care such as the recording of any allergies, relevant medical history and relevant obstetric issues. However, it is important that a 'tick box' application not be followed at all times and that topics be appropriately discussed according to the woman's needs. It is therefore important before using the questionnaires to ask if there are any particular topics that the woman herself wants to discuss. This may lead to a conversation that is led by the woman and not guided by the institutional questionnaires. Creating such space that allows the woman to speak and be heard may elucidate information that may otherwise may be omitted completely.

- Medical history – Explain that this part of the appointment is to clarify any medical history or underlying medical conditions that may impact on health during the pregnancy and that, if any are identified, referral to an obstetrician is the recommended pathway for care (Keeping Childbirth Natural and Dynamic [KCND] 2009) and is recommended for safety reasons.
- Social history, including living arrangements, significant family support and whether the woman smokes, drinks alcohol excessively or takes illicit street drugs. These are more potentially difficult conversations because, depending on living arrangements or

social situation, referral to social workers may be indicated. The individual's weight should be discussed during this part of the conversation; however, wherever it is raised in the conversation, one must be mindful of language and use terminology that is acceptable and easily understood. As discussed in the introduction, the words 'weight' and 'overweight' have been found to be the most acceptable to individuals (Brown & Flint 2021).

> I've identified that you weight is high, I'd like to discuss this in more detail with you. This is so that together we can discuss how to optimise your health during your pregnancy; this may mean that, after discussion, I refer you to an obstetrician at the hospital. Is that acceptable to you?

Raising the topic of unhealthy weight may elicit negative responses, as discussed above. Allow the individual a few minutes before proceeding, validate her feelings and then proceed in a positive manner:

> I can see you are surprised/disappointed by me telling you that you are overweight and that this may cause complications during your pregnancy. However, we know that improving diet, engaging in physical activity and stabilising your weight during pregnancy can improve health for women and babies. Can we discuss this further?

When the woman and her family members are ready, explain what the risks are to her and her baby when living with obesity but be cautious; at this stage, it may be wise to ask what the woman wants to know and ascertain what she already does know about the potential complications of living with an unhealthy weight. Too much information about life-threatening conditions such as deep vein thrombosis (DVT) and pre-eclampsia may be too much for some at this early stage in the relationship, so information should be moderated according to the woman's needs. It may also be the case that the woman will decline information. If this is the case, accept it and inform her that you will document the discussion in the records and that you would like to revisit this at a later time in the pregnancy.

Information, Motivation and Behaviour Change

In healthcare, providing information is second nature; we regularly inform people about procedures and medications and give the underpinning rationales for various procedures. However, providing information alone does not guarantee that individuals will act on that information and change their behaviour. Therefore, after the individual is informed of the health concern (in this case, unhealthy weight), something else needs to occur during the conversation that might motivate and support people to alter their habits.

Motivational interviewing (MI) is described as a form of interviewing where the individual is regarded by the interviewer with positive regard with the objective of facilitating the interviewee to examine negative behaviours and change their course of action (Tober & Raistrick 2007). Educational programmes are available for professionals to become qualified in this specific type of interviewing. However, one can draw on the principles of MI and, together with the individual, explore with them why they choose unhealthy foods or eat too much of it, for example; this, in turn, may allow them to identify what the triggers are for making such choices and consider how they might moderate them in the future. A similar approach can be taken when discussing physical activity. The theory that underpins this approach is that the individual's self-efficacy will be 'tapped' into, which will develop self-belief and in turn behaviour change (Moss 2017). However, discussing risk and asking people to change behaviours to mitigate risk aren't enough, and one should always provide achievable advice and ensure ongoing support of any behaviour change endeavours (Furness et al. 2011).

Antenatal appointments are time-constrained and are not designed for lengthy discussions such as the ones suggested above. However, maternity care takes place over several months, during which supportive relationships are developed between the woman, her family and the professional; therefore, it is likely that, over time, opportunities will arise and meaningful discussion can be facilitated with the aim of supporting the woman to change behaviours that in turn will promote her health and that of her unborn baby. With the changing shape of maternity car provision in the UK to a 'Continuity of Care' (CoC) model (NHS England 2017; Scottish government 2017), the ability of midwives to personalise the woman's journey and offer additional antenatal appointments that meet the woman's needs should be considered.

Closing the Encounter (Summarising and Planning)

Both the Calgary-Cambridge (2013) model of consultation and the Meitter & Karnieli-Miller (2021) model maintain that, after discussion about the problem or imparting the bad or sensitive issue, summarising what has been said and planning for the future are important. It will therefore be important to recap what has been discussed and ensure that the individual understands what will happen next.

- Ask the woman if she understands what has been discussed and if she has any additional questions.
- Make a contract (Silverman et al. 2013). Ensure that there is clarity between the woman and the professional about what the ongoing plan is – next appointments and any referrals to external agencies – and reiterate what will optimise the woman's health in terms of diet and exercise.
- Reiterate that weight loss is not what is advised during pregnancy.
- Reassure that the advice that has been provided with respect to diet and physical activity is evidence-based and that when attention is given to positive lifestyle changes, pregnancy outcomes can be optimised, but also remember to provide achievable advice.
- Provide appropriate public health information literature with oral explanation about its value.

Following the Appointment – Critical Reflection

Becoming a critically reflective practitioner is a professional expectation (NMC 2019); furthermore, Meitter & Karnieli-Miller (2021) advocate for this after a difficult consultation and suggest that it is necessary for professional growth and development. Therefore, following such a challenging encounter (if it has been so), take time, using a reflective model such as the Gibbs (1988), to formally reflect up on the episode. Consider how it has made you feel, how you consider that you performed and how you would repeat a similar session.

Documentation

Documentation is a fundamental part of healthcare and serves several purposes (Symon 2017; Kerkin et al. 2018); it makes professional work 'visible', is a means of communicating with colleagues and is a recording of the events that have occurred during a care episode. We have professional and legal obligations to maintain accurate records with respect to the care we have provided, the conversations that we have had and the care that we plan for individuals (Symon 2017). Currently, it is often tempting to document 'as we go'; whilst this may feel like we are being time-efficient, we may be missing important non-verbal cues. The Code (NMC 2018) suggests that records be documented at the end of a care episode. However, the practicalities of this during a clinic appointment may be difficult to achieve when one is faced with a 'tick box' questionnaire; it is also important that women be aware of what is written about them. Whether documentation occurs during or following the encounter, it should be thorough and contain a rationale as to why decisions have been made, and the professional must ensure that the woman is aware of what has been written about her. If using electronic records, then make use of 'free text' boxes and detail the conversations that have taken place. This provides information for others who may meet the woman at future dates as to what has been discussed and serves as an aide-mémoire for oneself when meeting the same person during subsequent encounters.

Conclusion

This chapter has considered the value of using structured consultation models to construct antenatal conversations, moving away from the 'tick box' format of using

Box 1.1 Professional Reflective Questions

- In the course of your practice, consider how you structure antenatal appointments.
  - What guides your dialogue?
  - How much do you veer away from prescriptive questionnaires?
  - How might making use of formal consultation models in the future support your professional practice?
- Consider how much preparation, if any, you give to your emotional preparation for an antenatal appointment where you may have to discuss sensitive topics.
  - How do you think you will proceed in the future with respect to emotional preparation prior to an appointment?
  - Consider what the benefits of preparing emotionally might be for both you and the pregnant woman.
- Consider how often you critically reflect upon your practice.
  - What model of reflection will most suit your needs when reflecting upon your antenatal skills?
  - What aspects of your consultation skills do you believe could be strengthened?
- Consider a recent consultation episode that you have facilitated and formally reflect upon it.
  - What have you learnt about yourself and your consultation skills?
  - What, if anything, might you do differently in a similar context?

institutional questionnaires. It has considered how utilising such a structured approach might facilitate a discussion about living with an unhealthy weight. A suggestion for constructing the consultation has been provided that combines the Calgary-Cambridge consultation model and the Meitter & Karnieli model for breaking bad news. Drawing on the principles of MI to support people to change their behaviour has also been considered. Having read this chapter, please now consider answers to the questions posed in Box 1.1.

Note

1 It is understood that for some, interpretation services may be required.

References

Bharj, K. K., & Daniels, L. (2017). Confirming pregnancy and care of the pregnant woman. In S. Macdonald & G. Johnson (Eds.), *Mayes' Midwifery* (15th ed.). Elsevier.

Brown, A., & Flint, S. W. (2021). Preferences and emotional response to weight-related terminology used by healthcare professionals to describe body weight in people living with overweight and obesity. *Clinical Obesity*, *11*(5). https://doi.org/10.1111/cob.12470

Chan, S. W., Tulloch, E., Cooper, E. S., Smith, A., Wojcik, W., & Norman, J. E. (2017). Montgomery and informed consent: Where are we now? *BMJ (Online)*, *357*, j2224–j2224. https://doi.org/10.1136/bmj.j2224

Denison, F. C., Aedla, N. R., Keag, O., Hor, K., Reynolds, R. M., Milne, A., Diamond, A., Amir, L., Bodnar, L. M., Beckett, V., Bouch, C., Cousins, J., Duckitt, K., Fox, K. A., Fraser, D., McCurdy, R. J., Salama, H., Salama, H. S., Smith, G. C. S., ... Thomson, A. J. (2018). Care of women with obesity in pregnancy green-top guideline no. 72. *BJOG: An International Journal of Obstetrics and Gynaecology*, *126*(3), E62–E106. https://doi.org/10.1111/1471-0528.15386

Denness, C. (2013). What are consultation models for? *InnovAiT*, *6*(9), 592–599. https://doi.org/10.1177/1755738013475436

Furness, J., McSeveny, K., Arden, M. A., Garland, C., Dearden, A. M., & Soltani, H. (2011). Maternal obesity support services: a qualitative study of the perspectives of women and midwives. *BMC Pregnancy and Childbirth*, *11*(1), 69–69. https://doi.org/10.1186/1471-2393-11-69

Gibbs, G (1988). *Learning by Doing: A guide to teaching and learning methods*. Further Education Unit. Oxford Polytechnic, Oxford.

Granger, K. (2014). Hello My Name Is. YouTube. Retrieved from https://www.youtube.com/watch?v=UmeQjgy4QnE

Greig, Y., Williams, A. F., & Coulter-Smith, M. (2021). Obesity matters: The skills that strengthen midwifery practice when caring for obese pregnant women. *British Journal of Midwifery*, *29*(5), 278–285. https://doi.org/10.12968/bjom.2021.29.5.278

Health Improvement Scotland. (2009). Keeping Childbirth Natural and Dynamic: Pathways for maternity care. Retrieved 3rd December 2023, from https://www.healthcareimprovementscotland.org/our_work/reproductive,_maternal_child/programme_resources/keeping_childbirth_natural.asp

Heslehurst, N., Russell, S., McCormack, S., Sedgewick, G., Bell, R., & Rankin, J. (2013). Midwives perspectives of their training and education requirements in maternal obesity: A qualitative study. *Midwifery*, *29*(7), 736–744. https://doi.org/10.1016/j.midw.2012.07.007

Jomeen, J. (2017). Psychological context of childbirth. In S. Macdonald & G. Johnson (Eds.), *Mayes' Midwifery* (15th ed., pp. 186–199). Elsevier.

Kerkin, B., Lennox, S., & Patterson, J. (2018). Making midwifery work visible: The multiple purposes of documentation. *Women and Birth: Journal of the Australian College of Midwives*, *31*(3), 232–239. https://doi.org/10.1016/j.wombi.2017.09.012

Knight Agarwal, C. R., Kaur, M., Williams, L. T., Davey, R., & Davis, D. (2014). The views and attitudes of health professionals providing antenatal care to women with a high BMI: A qualitative research study. *Women and Birth*, 27(1), 138–144. https://doi.org/10.1016/j.wombi.2013.11.002

Launer, J. (2018). *Narrative-based practiced in health and social care. Conversations inviting change.* (2nd ed.). Routledge.

McParlin, C., et al. (2017). What helps or hinders midwives to implement physical activity guidelines for obese pregnant women? A questionnaire survey using the theoretical domains framework. *Midwifery*, 49, 110–116.

Meitter, D., & Karnieli-Miller, O. (2021). Twelve tips to manage a breaking bad news process: Using SPw-ICE-S–A revised version of the SPIKES protocol. *Medical Teacher*, 1–5. https://doi.org/10.1080/0142159X.2021.1928618

Moss, B. (2017). *Communication skills in health and social care* (4th ed.). SAGE.

Neighbour, R. (2005). *The inner consultation, how to develop an effective and intuitive consultation style* (2nd ed.). CRC Press.

NHS England. (2017). *Better Births: Improving outcomes of maternity services in England – A five year forward view for maternity care.* Retrieved 28, November, from https://www.england.nhs.uk/publication/better-births-improving-outcomes-of-maternity-services-in-england-a-five-year-forward-view-for-maternity-care/

Nursing and Midwifery Council. (2018). *The code: Professional standards of practice and behaviour for nurses, midwives and nursing associates.* Retrieved from https://www.nmc.org.uk/search/?q=The+code

Nursing and Midwifery Council. (2019). *Standards of proficiency for midwives.* Retrieved from https://www.nmc.org.uk/standards/standards-for-midwives/standards-of-proficiency-for-midwives/

Scottish Government. (2017). The Best Start: five-year plan for maternity and neonatal care. Retrieved 28, November, from https://www.gov.scot/publications/best-start-five-year-forward-plan-maternity-neonatal-care-scotland/

Silverman, J., Kurrz, S., & Draper, J. (2013). Skills for communicating with patients (3rd ed.). Radcliffe publishing.

Symon, A. (2017). The law and the midwife. In S. Macdonald & G. Johnson (Eds), Mayes' Midwifery (15th ed., pp 139–157). Elsevier.

The Best Start: Five Year Plan for Maternity and Neonatal Care. (2017). The Scottish government 2017 (Online). Retrieved 7 April 2019, from https://www.gov.scot/publications/best-start-five-year-forward-plan-maternity-neonatal-carescotland

Tober, G., & Raistrick, D. (2007). *Motivational dialogue: Preparing addiction professionals for motivational interviewing practice.* Routledge.

Witt, K., & Jorgensen, M. (2016). *The logic and chronology of consultations in general practice - Teaching consultation skills in medical school.* MedEdPublish. https://doi.org/10.15694/mep.2016.000111

2 Health Risks and Complications for Women

Introduction

Chapter 1 discussed in some detail *how* to construct a consultation episode. However, being knowledgeable about consultation construction is only part of the professional narrative; having a clear understanding about the potential complications a woman may face and the underlying pathophysiology that living with excessive adipose tissue causes is also required if we are to provide thorough and evidence-based information for her and her family. This chapter discusses some of the health complications that may arise for women and their unborn babies during pregnancy when they live with an unhealthy weight. It includes an overview of the functions of adipose tissue and explains why living with an excess amount of this tissue type increases the potential health risks for women.

Whilst reading this chapter, one should, however, be cognisant that the risk of these complications arising increases with both the level of obesity and maternal age. This is significant because the average age of first-time mothers in the UK is now 30–39 years (Office for National Statistics 2020). Although the age of a woman and her pre-pregnancy weight may place her at increased risk of altered health, it must be borne in mind that some 37% of obese women will encounter no problems and go on to have uneventful pregnancies and deliver a healthy baby.

The Role of Adipose Tissue and 'Metabolic Syndrome'

Metabolic syndrome is understood to be a collection of physiological, biochemical and metabolic factors that non-pregnant individuals who live with an unhealthy weight may encounter. It is a collective term for conditions such as cardiovascular disease, type 2 diabetes mellitus (T2DM), insulin resistance, raised blood pressure (BP), chronic inflammation and a reduction in the body's ability to fight infection (Kaur 2014; Ellulu et al. 2017). Non-pregnant individuals who live with an unhealthy weight are at risk of developing any or all of these conditions; and if they do, this may severely impact their ongoing health. When a woman who is already obese, and who may already be living with some of these conditions, becomes pregnant, further risk is superimposed on her health and that of her unborn baby.

There is now evidence that white adipose tissue (WAT) is not an inert substance; rather, it behaves as an endocrine organ-secreting hormone such as leptin and renin (Ellulu et al. 2017); renin secreted from abdominal fat has been associated with hypertension in obese

DOI: 10.4324/9781003332398-3

individuals (Clancy & McVicar 2009). Leptin is a hormone that regulates appetite, but when it's produced in large amounts, 'leptin resistance' occurs and leads to dysregulated appetite and excessive eating (Ellulu et al. 2017).

Excessive macrophage production is also seen in the adipose tissue (Blokhin & Lentz 2013; Ellulu et al. 2017) and causes chronic low-grade inflammation that predisposes individuals to cardiovascular disease, hypertension, and venous thromboembolytic (VTE) disease. Concurrently, there is also a decrease in the production of anti-coagulant factors and increased production of thrombin-enhanced platelet activity (Blokhin & Lentz 2013), which increases the risk of developing VTE disease.

The secretion of adipokines (cell-signalling proteins) from the adipose tissue is thought to cause insulin resistance. The term 'insulin resistance' is used to describe how the body does not respond effectively to one of the glucose-regulating hormones, 'insulin,' leading to the body's inability to dispose of excessive glucose; this leads to a rise in blood glucose levels and predisposes the individual to T2DM (Hardy et al. 2012).

Pregnant women who are obese may present for maternity care having never seen a medical professional for many years and may be in the early stages of developing metabolic syndrome, or indeed they may already have developed some signs and symptoms that have not previously been diagnosed. This means that midwives must be vigilant in screening, risk-assessing and monitoring those who live with unhealthy weights and be clear about what they tell women with respect to the health risks that they may encounter as the pregnancy progresses and how to mitigate them.

Dysregulated Appetite

During pregnancy, appetite can be affected by commonly seen nausea and vomiting or, in extreme cases, hyperemesis gravidarum (HG). However, when these symptoms of pregnancy eventually settle, it is possible that an excessive appetite will resume, meaning that the woman may continue to gain excessive weight throughout the pregnancy. Where there has been excessive nausea or vomiting or HG, women should have their weight monitored. Whilst reducing the body mass index (BMI) may bring general health benefits, rapid weight loss during pregnancy can be harmful to both mother and baby; the mother can become malnourished, and the developing baby is at risk of growth restriction (Jewell 2017). Therefore, if, on monitoring, weight loss is found to have been rapid, even when the BMI is raised, referral to obstetricians should also be made to ensure appropriate surveillance and management of the woman's health during the remainder of her pregnancy.

Miscarriage

Miscarriage is defined as a pregnancy that ends prior to 24 completed weeks of pregnancy where the foetus is not alive (Hutcherson 2017).

Whilst it is understood that early miscarriage may be due to chromosomal abnormality, obesity has been identified as an independent risk factor for pregnancy loss, including stillbirth and miscarriage (Malasevskaia et al. 2021). In addition, they concluded that living with a raised BMI had a negative effect on a woman's "oocytes, embryos and hormones" and acknowledged that further endocrine research was required to fully understand the biochemical mechanisms that can lead to a failed pregnancy. This suggests that women who live with an unhealthy weight may not find it easy to conceive in the first place, and this, in turn, may lead to heightened anxiety levels for them during pregnancy when they do conceive, especially if they are made aware of the possible complications that obesity can predispose them to. For some who have suffered pregnancy loss, engagement in physical activity may be anxiety-provoking or considered dangerous in pregnancy for the baby, meaning that it is reduced or avoided altogether. However, avoiding physical activity can further compound the pregnancy and increase the risk yet again of complications arising (discussed in Chapter 5).

Cavalcante et al. (2019) identified that obese women were at increased risk of suffering from recurrent pregnancy losses. Miscarriage can be a devastating experience for women and their families and can result in a prolonged grief reaction and, in some cases, post-traumatic stress disorder (PTSD). For women who have suffered recurrent miscarriages (three consecutive losses), anxiety is likely to be amplified, highlighting the need for midwives to provide accurate advice about weight-related complications and how to mitigate them. These conversations need to be meaningful and compassionate whilst providing positive advice about how to optimise and protect health throughout their maternity care journey and beyond.

Gestational Diabetes

Gestational diabetes mellitus (GDM) is a condition unique to pregnancy and results in hyperglycaemia due to an impaired carbohydrate metabolic pathway (Bothamley & Boyle 2017). This is driven by placental hormones that ensure the body stores sufficient carbohydrates contributing to foetal growth and that provide the pregnant body with energy for labour, birth and breastfeeding (Bothamley & Boyle 2017).

The risk of an obese pregnant women developing GDM has been found to rise depending upon the category of obesity (class I, class II or class III) (Chu et al. 2007). Gestational diabetes is associated with adverse pregnancy outcomes such as foetal anomaly, preterm birth or stillbirth (Bothamley & Boyle 2017; Denison et al. 2018); Ali & Dornhurst 2018).

Current national guidance suggests that all women who present for care in the UK with a BMI of at least 30 kg/m^2 should be screened for gestational diabetes (Denison et al., 2018). This may cause tension for some midwives as they strive to operate within a philosophy that is underpinned by 'normality'. However, women have a right to be informed about potential complications they may face with respect to dysregulated glycaemic control. A detailed discussion about the risk of developing GDM, its potential complications as well as any additional monitoring that would be offered must be undertaken, and midwives should be cognisant of their professional obligations (Nursing and Midwifery Council [NMC] 2018, 2019). It is, however, the woman's decision as to whether she accepts or declines any additional screening that is offered, and she needs to make an informed decision about whether to accept an oral glucose tolerance test or not.

If GDM is diagnosed, the woman will require care from a multi-disciplinary team: midwives, obstetricians, diabetologists, diabetic specialist nurses and dietitians. She must be made aware that this diagnosis places her at 'high risk,' and she has a right to know what these risks are.

She must also be made aware that postnatally she will be offered further investigations to ensure that her diabetic status has resolved. If her status has not resolved, it is likely that she has developed T2DM, and this will require ongoing diabetic care and management.

Hypertension

Hypertension is a recognised risk for obese individuals who are not pregnant (National Institute for Health and Care Excellence [NICE] 2019a; Seravalle & Grassi 2017). If an obese individual becomes pregnant, they are super-imposing the risk of pregnancy complications onto an already 'at risk' body, especially if they are found to have undiagnosed essential hypertension on presentation for maternity care.

Essential hypertension is defined as a raised BP between 140/90 mm Hg and 180/120 mm Hg (NICE 2019b) that is detected in an asymptomatic individual. For some women, pregnancy may be the first time they have ever had their BP measured and so to learn that it is already raised may be anxiety-provoking. Depending upon the level of the raised BP, referral should be made for medical review; in some cases, anti-hypertension medication may be prescribed early in the pregnancy.

Pre-eclampsia and eclampsia are multi-system diseases that are unique to pregnancy (Bothamley & Boyle 2017; Waugh & Smith 2018). These conditions are caused by abnormal implantation of the placenta very early in the pregnancy and are typically characterised by seeing a raised BP (≥140/90 mm Hg), excessive oedema and cerebral oedema resulting in blurred vision and frontal headaches, altered renal function and, in cases of eclampsia, seizures (Bothamley & Boyle 2017). When superimposed upon essential hypertension, diagnosing pre-eclampsia can be challenging (Waugh & Smith 2018). Knight et al. (2021) have cited hypertensive disease of pregnancy as being a dominant cause of maternal death in the UK.

Superimposing a pregnancy on an already hypertensive body increases the risk of developing pre-eclampsia and eclampsia and, in turn, risks the health of the mother or unborn baby or both. Accurate monitoring of BP during pregnancy is a central part of midwifery practice performed at every interaction during the childbirth journey, but often errors are made in measuring this accurately because of an inappropriately sized BP cuff being used (Denison et al., 2018; Waugh & Smith 2018). Using the correct and appropriate equipment is essential if errors are to be minimised. The size of a BP cuff used for obese people is large and is labelled a 'thigh cuff.' For some women, seeing such a large cuff may cause distress; therefore, a carefully-thought-out explanation and rationale should be given when using specialist equipment. If essential hypertension is diagnosed early in pregnancy, the woman will require a senior medical review and such a referral will also need to be carefully explained.

Current guidance from the Denison et al. (2018) suggests that where women have specific risk factors for developing pre-eclampsia, taking aspirin 75 mg daily may mitigate them. Obese women at risk of developing pre-eclampsia therefore are advised to follow this pathway. However, taking medication in pregnancy for 'no reason' may be unacceptable to some women, necessitating careful discussion and explanation as to its benefits.

Venous Thromboembolytic (VTE) Disease

VTE disease is now the fourth most common cause of maternal death (Knight et al. 2021), and those who survive a VTE episode can suffer significant ongoing morbidity. There are three components of thrombus formation: static blood, hypercoagulability, and blood vessel wall damage (Davis & Pavord 2018). During pregnancy, an increase in coagulation factors and relaxation of the venous walls (as a result of high progesterone levels) weaken blood vessel walls and increase the risk of blood 'pooling' in the veins of the lower limbs (Coad et al. 2020); all increase the risk of developing VTE disease. The absolute risk of developing VTE is low for all pregnancies (1:1000) (Davis & Pavord 2018). However, when the BMI is at least 30 kg/m^2, the risk of developing VTE disease is increased; furthermore, a raised BMI has been identified as an independent risk factor for recurrent VTE episodes.

It is worth noting here that whilst many women are well following pregnancy and birth, some suffer from significant morbidity during the post-partum period (Davis & Pavord 2018; Bick et al. 2020). Careful explanation about this must be provided and the woman must be informed during her pregnancy that she may receive low-molecular-weight heparin (LMWH) 'blood thinning' injections to self-administer following birth to reduce the risk of developing VTE Denison et al., (2018) postnatally.

Prolonged pregnancy and increased chance of Caesarean section

Women who are obese are at greater risk of having a pregnancy that progresses beyond forty weeks' gestation (Bogaerts et al. 2013), meaning that they are at risk of requiring induction of labour (IOL) with the incumbent risks of using prostaglandins and oxytocin to establish or augment labour or both (Jordan & Macdonald 2017). When women do experience spontaneous uterine contractions, there appears to be dysfunction in the myometrium and an altered contraction pattern can be observed as a result of raised adiposity (Bogaerts et al. 2013). Requiring IOL beyond forty weeks and ten days increases the risk of requiring delivery by Caesarean section (C/S) for all woman, but this risk is increased when women live with an unhealthy weight (Bogaerts et al., 2013). This may be attributed to the disruption of hormonal balance that obese women encounter and to increased secretion of adipokines from adipose tissue (Azaïs et al. 2017).

Obese women who ultimately require delivery by C/S are therefore at increased risk of developing post-operative complications such as wound, chest and urinary infections, pressure sores and VTE disease due to immobility and in general of having a longer and more prolonged recovery than those of normal weight (Bassett 2017). The woman should be advised that if she gives birth as a result of operative delivery, she is at increased risk of the post-operative complications mentioned above.

Post-Partum Haemorrhage

Post-partum haemorrhage (PPH) is associated with a BMI of at least 30 kg/m^2, and active management of the third stage is recommended (Denison et al. 2018). However, it is likely that this risk will be attributable to the obstetric interventions themselves, such as IOL with vaginal prostaglandins, prolonged labour due to uterine dysfunction, augmentation of labour with intravenous oxytocin, and C/S required to provide safe care for women who live with an unhealthy weight rather than obesity itself (Chodanker et al. 2017; Davey et al. 2020).

PPH can be difficult to manage in obese individuals; the fundus can be difficult to palpate, causing delay in manually stimulating a contraction, and if IV access hasn't been established, this may also be challenging. Administering a significant amount of medication may be required to bring any bleeding under control. Ultimately, obese women who suffer from major obstetric haemorrhage may need to be examined in theatre under anaesthesia, leading to further risks of immobility and a long recovery. This eventuality is also likely to separate mother and baby, causing anxiety for her and her family.

Adversely Affected Mental Health

There is now clear evidence that women who are obese are much more likely to suffer from a range of mental health conditions that include anxiety, stress and depression both during the antenatal and postnatal periods (Molyneaux et al. 2016; Steinig et al., 2017; Salehi-Pourmehr et al. 2019). The absolute reasons for this are not fully understood, but Oskis (2022) explains that food and feelings are intermingled and that sugar can 'soothe' bad feelings, suggesting that when one feels low or sad, it is food that is turned to for comfort. Therefore, for some, poor mental health symptoms may already have been present prior to pregnancy, and obesity developed secondary to this as a result of overeating unhealthy foods; conversely, living with an unhealthy weight may have caused low mood. No matter the cause, however, midwives need to be aware that women who live with an unhealthy weight appear to be especially vulnerable to developing mental health illness.

Poor perinatal mental health that encompasses anxiety and depression as well as pre-existing illnesses such as bi-polar disorder and schizophrenia can lead to poor birth outcomes. Knight et al. (2021), have identified that suicide is now the leading cause of maternal death during the first year after pregnancy in the UK. Poor maternal mental health not only affects the mother both during and after pregnancy but also can be detrimental for foetal development and throughout the child's lifetime continuum (Caparros-Gonzalez et al. 2021). Research findings have also shown that the combination of poor maternal diet and maternal stress can play a part in atypical brain development of the foetus during pregnancy (Niculescu & Lupu 2009; Mina et al. 2017).

This may be a difficult topic to raise with women amongst the myriad of other topics that pertain to obesity. However, it is important for midwives to monitor women's psychological well-being carefully throughout pregnancy and in the postnatal period, noting any change in her mood or deterioration in her mental health. Developing continuity of care and carer as advocated in the driver documents (NHS England 2017; The Scottish Government 2017) will likely facilitate the building of a trusting relationship between the woman and the midwife and make it easier for the midwife to ask sensitive questions about her mental health or indeed to notice any changes in the woman's mental state. Ensuring early and appropriate referral to appropriate mental health services is fundamental in optimising the woman's ongoing health during her pregnancy.

Musculo-Skeletal Dysfunction and Pain

Pelvic girdle pain is a commonly seen difficulty for some pregnant women (Brook 2017). However, for those who are obese, it has been recognised for some years that the risk of this so-called 'minor' complication is increased (Denison et al. 2009). However, it is likely that women who suffer from this condition during pregnancy do not consider it 'minor' if it impacts negatively upon their quality of life. With increased pain, there is a risk that they may require increased oral analgesia that may include opioids, and depending on the medication used, this may lead to neonatal abstinence syndrome (NAS) in the newborn (Petty 2019). One can imagine that an expectant mother in such a situation will be anxious and have feelings of guilt that she may ultimately harm her baby.

Suffering from musculo-skeletal pain may also deter and, in some cases, preclude the woman from engaging in any physical activity. Being unable to exercise is likely to disrupt her weight management plans and risk her weight rising, further compounding the risks of obesity. Timely referral to an obstetric or women's health physiotherapy must be considered to ensure that optimal care and advice are provided to optimise the woman's mobility. Referral to obstetricians may also be necessary to ensure appropriate management of pain, to discuss the ongoing management plan during the pregnancy and to discuss a plan for giving birth because, in some cases, C/S is necessary.

Breastfeeding Challenges

Women who live with an unhealthy weight appear to have difficulty establishing and sustaining breastfeeding (Ballesta-Castillejos et al., 2020). This may be due to the physical challenges of attaching a very small baby to a large breast, and women who live with high levels of adiposity may not be able to observe well how they are positioning the baby on the breast or have difficulty in finding a comfortable position for them and their baby. However, Preusting et al. (2017) suggest that there are more physiological reasons for breastfeeding difficulties when a mother is obese. They observed that the onset of lactogenesis took longer for women who had a BMI of at least 30 kg/m^2 compared with their normal-weight counterparts: 85.2 hours compared with 72 hours, which is the 'normal' length of time for lactogenesis to occur (Preusting et al. 2017). Furthermore, Rasmussen and Kjolhede (2004) and Bever Babendure et al. (2015) noted that obese women appeared to have a reduced prolactin response when the baby suckled, meaning that there was likely to be a diminished milk supply. Another contributing factor pertaining to reduced lactation is that of insulin resistance. Recent evidence suggests that mature milk production is reliant upon insulin to ensure secretory activation (Nommsen-Rivers 2016), suggesting that women who are insulin-resistant, such as obese women, will have difficulty in establishing breastfeeding. The combination of physical difficulties of positioning, delayed lactogenesis, insulin resistance and poor prolactin response puts the baby at risk of not receiving enough breastmilk in the early days of life. This is likely to cause anxiety for women and can further interfere with the lactogenesis pathway and places the baby at risk of requiring formula supplementation.

Conclusion

This chapter has provided an overview of some of the most common complications that obese women may encounter during pregnancy. Women have the right to be informed about how their unhealthy weight may impact their health and that of their baby, how to mitigate such complications, and what screening tests are available for them and be provided with ongoing pregnancy management plans. Carefully designed conversations should be constructed so that relevant information is provided in a way that is comprehensible, meaningful and compassionate for individual women and should allow for the woman's voice to be heard too. Professionals need to be aware that discussing these topics may evoke negative responses that may be anxiety-provoking for women.

Discussing some of these issues will be inevitable in practice. Consider how you will develop your practice with respect to these potential complications by considering the questions in Box 2.1.

Box 2.1 Professional Reflective Questions

- Reflect upon your practice and consider some of the obese women whom you have provided care to.
  - Did they develop any of the above-mentioned complications during their pregnancy or birth or in the postnatal period?
  - Make a list of the complications they developed (if any).
  - Consider if the women that you are thinking about were aware of their increased risk in developing the complication.
- Now think about any consultations you may have observed medical staff discussing with obese women who have developed complications.
  - Were the medical staff honest in discussing complications?
  - Did they clearly explain the complications that had arisen?
  - What was the reaction of the woman (and her family members)? Shock? Surprise? Or did the woman appear to have been 'well prepared' for what might occur?
- Consider how you will practice with respect to discussing complications with an 'unprepared' woman.
  - Consider what language you will use (e.g., BMI, obesity, unhealthy weight).
  - What additional reading will you undertake?
  - Consider what advice you might provide with respect to the following:
    1. Current recovery?
    2. Future pregnancies?

References

Azaïs, H, Leroy, A., Ghesquiere, L., Deruelle, P., & Hanssens, S. (2017). Effects of adipokines and obesity on uterine contractility. *Cytokine & Growth Factor Reviews*, *34*, 59–66. https://doi.org/10.1016/j.cytogfr.2017.01.001

Ballesta-Castillejos, A., Gomez-Salgado, J., Rodriguez-Almagro, J., Ortiz-Esquinas, I., & Hernandez-Martinez, A. (2020). Relationship between maternal body mass index with the onset of breastfeeding and its associated problems: An online survey. *International Breastfeeding Journal*, *15*(1), 55–55. https://doi.org/10.1186/s13006-020-00298-5

Bassett, S. (2017). Obstetric interventions. In S. Macdonald & G. Johnson (Eds.), *Mayes' midwifery* (15th ed.). Elsevier.

Bever Babendure, J., Reifsnider, E., Mendias, E., Moramarco, M. W., & Davila, Y. R. (2015). Reduced breastfeeding rates among obese mothers: A review of contributing factors, clinical considerations and future directions. *International Breastfeeding Journal*, *10*(1), 21–21. https://doi.org/10.1186/s13006-015-0046-5

Bick, D., Duff, E., & Shakespeare, J. (2020). Better births – But why not better postnatal care? *Midwifery*, *80*, 102574. https://doi.org/10.1016/j.midw.2019.102574

Blokhin, I. O., & Lentz, S. R. (2013). Mechanisms of thrombosis in obesity. *Current opinion in hematology*, *20*(5), 437–444. https://doi.org/10.1097/MOH.0b013e3283634443

Bogaerts, A., Witters, I., Van den Bergh, B. R. H., Jans, G., & Devlieger, R. (2013). Obesity in pregnancy: Altered onset and progression of labour. *Midwifery*, 29(12), 1303–1313. https://doi.org/10.1016/j.midw.2012.12.013

Bothamley, J., & Boyle, M. 2017. Hypertensive and medical disorders in pregnancy. In S. Macdonald & G. Johnson (Eds.), *Mayes' midwifery* (15th ed.). Elsevier.

Brook, G. (2017). Physical preparation for childbirth and beyond: The role of physiotherapy. In. S. Macdonald & G. Johnson (Eds.), *Mayes' midwifery* (15th ed.). Elsevier.

Caparros-Gonzalez, R. A., Torre-Luque, A. d. L., Romero-Gonzalez, B., Quesada-Soto, J. M., Alderdice, F., & Peralta-Ramírez, M. I. (2021). Stress during pregnancy and the development of diseases in the offspring: A systematic-review and meta-analysis. *Midwifery*, *97*, 102939. https://doi.org/10.1016/j.midw.2021.102939

Cavalcante, M. B., Sarno, M., Peixoto, A. B., Araujo Júnior, E., & Barini, R. (2019). Obesity and recurrent miscarriage: A systematic review and meta-analysis. *Journal of Obstetrics and Gynaecology Research*, *45*(1), 30–38. https://doi.org/10.1111/jog.13799

Chodanker, R., Middleton, G., Linn, C., & Mahmood, T. (2017). Obesity in pregnancy. *Obstetrics, Gynaecology and Reproductive Medicine*, *28*(2). https://doi.org/10.1016/j.ogrm.2017.11.003

Chu, S. Y., Callaghan, W. M., Kim, S. Y., Schmid, C. H., Lau, J., England, L. J., & Dietz, P. M. (2007). Maternal obesity and risk of gestational diabetes mellitus. *Diabetes Care*, *30*(8), 2070–2076. https://doi.org/10.2337/dc06-2559a

Clancy, J., & McVicar, A. J. (2009). *Physiology and anatomy for nurses and healthcare practitioners: a homeostatic approach* (3rd ed.). Hodder Arnold.

Coad, J., Pedley, K., & Dunstall, M. (2020). *Anatomy and physiology for midwives* (4th ed.). Elsevier.

Davey, Flood M., Pollock, W., Cullinane, F., & McDonald, S. (2020). Risk factors for severe postpartum haemorrhage: A population-based retrospective cohort study. *Australian & New Zealand Journal of Obstetrics & Gynaecology*, *60*(4), 522–532. https://doi.org/10.1111/ajo.13099

Davis, S., & Pavord, S. (2018). Haematological problems in pregnancy. In Christoph Lees & Tom Bourne (Eds.), *Dewhurst's textbook of obstetrics and gynaecology*. John Wiley & Sons, Incorporated. Retrieved ProQuest Ebook Central, from https://ebookcentral.proquest.com/lib/nhsscotland-ebooks/detail.action?docID=5516881

Denison, F., Norrie, G., Graham, B., Lynch, J., Harper, N., & Reynolds, R. (2009). Increased maternal BMI is associated with an increased risk of minor complications during pregnancy with consequent cost implications. *BJOG: An International Journal of Obstetrics and Gynaecology*, *116*(11), 1467–1472. https://doi.org/10.1111/j.1471-0528.2009.02222.x

Denison, F. C., Aedla, N. R., Keag, O., Hor, K., Reynolds, R. M., Milne, A., & Diamond, A., (2018). Care of women with obesity in pregnancy. [NG72]. Green-top Guideline. On behalf of the Royal College of Obstetricians and Gynaecologists. Retrieved from https://www.rcog.org.uk/guidance/browse-all-guidance/green-top-guidelines/care-of-women-with-obesity-in-pregnancy-green-top-guideline-no-72/

Ellulu, M. S., Patimah, I., Khaza'ai, H., Rahmat, A., & Abed, Y. (2017). Obesity and inflammation: The linking mechanism and the complications. *Archives of Medical Science*, *13*(4), 851–863. https://doi.org/10.5114/aoms.2016.58928

Hardy, O. T., Czech, M. P., & Corvera, S. (2012). What causes the insulin resistance underlying obesity? *Current Opinion in Endocrinology, Diabetes, and Obesity*, *19*(2), 81–87. https://doi.org/10.1097/MED.0b013e3283514e13

Hutcherson, A., 2017. Bleeding in pregnancy. In S. Macdonald & G. Johnson (Eds.), *Mayes' midwifery* (15th ed.). Elsevier.

Jewell, K. (2017). Nutrition. In S. Macdonald & G. Johnson (Eds.), *Mayes' midwifery* (15th ed., pp. 262–287). Elsevier.

Jordan, S., & Macdonald, S. (2017). Pharmacology and the midwife. In S. Macdonald & G. Johnson (Eds.), *Mayes' midwifery*. (15th ed.). Elsevier.

Kaur, J. (2014). A comprehensive review on metabolic syndrome. *Cardiology Research and Practice*. https://doi.org/10.1155/2014/943162

Knight, M., Bunch, K., Tuffnell, D., Patel, R., Shakespeare, J., Kotnis, R., Kenyon, S., & Kurinczuk, J. J. (Eds.). (2021). Saving lives, improving mothers' care, lessons learned to inform maternity care from the UK and Ireland confidential enquiries into maternal deaths and morbidity 2017–19. *MBRACCE-UK*. Retrieved from https://www.npeu.ox.ac.uk/assets/downloads/mbrrace-uk/reports/maternal-report-2021/MBRRACE-UK_Maternal_Report_2021_-_FINAL_-_WEB_VERSION.pdf

Malasevskaia, I., Sultana, S., Hassan, A., Hafez, A. A., Onal, F., Ilgun, H., & Heindl, S. E. (2021). A 21st century epidemic-obesity: And its impact on pregnancy loss. *Cureus*, *13*(1), e12417. https://doi.org/10.7759/cureus.12417

Mina, T. H., Lahti, M., Drake, A. J., Räikkönen, K., Minnis, H., Denison, F. C., … Reynolds, R. M. (2017). Prenatal exposure to very severe maternal obesity is associated with adverse neuropsychiatric outcomes in children. *Psychological Medicine*, 47(2), 353–362. https://doi.org/10.1017/S0033291716002452

Molyneaux, E., Poston, L., Khondoker, M., & Howard, L. M. (2016). Obesity, antenatal depression, diet and gestational weight gain in a population cohort study. *Archives of Women's Mental Health*, *19*(5), 899–907. https://doi.org/10.1007/s00737-016-0635-3

National Institute for Health and Care Excellence. (2019a). Hypertension in adults: Diagnosis and management. Retrieved from https://www.nice.org.uk/guidance/ng136

National Institute for Health and Care Excellence. (2019b). Hypertension in adults: Diagnosis and management. [updated 2023]. Retrieved 3rd December 2023, from https://www.nice.org.uk/guidance/ng136

NHS England. (2017). *Better births: Improving outcomes of maternity services in England – A five year forward view for maternity care*. Retrieved from https://www.england.nhs.uk/publication/better-births-improving-outcomes-of-maternity-services-in-england-a-five-year-forward-view-for-maternity-care/

Niculescu, M. D., & Lupu, D. S. (2009). High fat diet-induced maternal obesity alters fetal hippocampal development. *International Journal of Developmental Neuroscience: The Official Journal of the International Society for Developmental Neuroscience*, 27(7), 627–633. https://doi.org/10.1016/j.ijdevneu.2009.08.005

Nommsen-Rivers, L. A. (2016). Does insulin explain the relation between maternal obesity and poor lactation outcomes? An overview of the literature. *Advances in Nutrition (Bethesda, Md.)*, 7(2), 407–414. https://doi.org/10.3945/an.115.011007

Nursing and Midwifery Council. (2018). *The code. Professional standards of practice and behaviour for nurses, midwives and nursing associates*. Retrieved from https://www.nmc.org.uk/standards/code/B

Nursing and Midwifery Council. (2019). *Standards of proficiency for midwives*. Retrieved from https://www.nmc.org.uk/standards/standards-for-midwives/standards-of-proficiency-for-midwives/

Office For National Statistics. (2020). *Tackling obesity: Government strategy*. UK Government. Retrieved from https://www.gov.uk/government/publications/tackling-obesity-government-strategy

Oskis, A. (2022). Food and feelings. In L. Cundy (Ed.), *Attachment, relationships and food: From cradle to kitchen* (pp. 40–57). Routledge.

Petty, J. (2019). *Bedside guide for neonatal care*. Macmillan International.

Preusting, I., Brumley, J., Odibo, L., Spatz, D. L., & Louis, J. M. (2017). Obesity as a predictor of delayed lactogenesis II. *Journal of Human Lactation*, *33*(4), 684–691. https://doi.org/10.1177/0890334417727716

Rasmussen, K. M., & Kjolhede, C. L. (2004). Prepregnant overweight and obesity diminish the prolactin response to suckling in the first week postpartum. *Pediatrics (Evanston)*, *113*(5), e465–e471. https://doi.org/10.1542/peds.113.5.e465

Salehi-Pourmehr, H., Dolatkhah, N., Gassab-Abdollahi, N., Farrin, N., Mojtahedi, M., & Farshbaf-Khalili, A. (2019). Screening of depression in overweight and obese pregnant women and its predictors. *Journal of Obstetrics and Gynaecology Research*, *45*(11), 2169–2177. https://doi.org/10.1111/jog.14100

Scottish Government. (2017). *The best start. A five year forward plan for maternity and neonatal care in Scotland.* Retrieved from https://www.gov.scot/binaries/content/documents/govscot/publications/strategy-plan/2017/01/best-start-five-year-forward-plan-maternity-neonatal-care-scotland/documents/00513175-pdf/00513175-pdf/govscot%3Adocument/00513175.pdf

Seravalle, G., & Grassi, G. (2017). Obesity and hypertension. *Pharmacological Research, 122*, 1–7. https://doi.org/10.1016/j.phrs.2017.05.013

Steinig, J., Nagl, M., Linde, K., Zietlow, G., & Kersting, A. (2017). Antenatal and postnatal depression in women with obesity: A systematic review. *Archives of Women's Mental Health, 20*(4), 569–585. https://doi.org/10.1007/s00737-017-0739-4

Waugh, J. J. S., & Smith, M. C. (2018). Hypertensive disorders. In Christoph Lees & Tom Bourne (Eds.), *Dewhurst's textbook of obstetrics and gynaecology.* John Wiley & Sons, Incorporated, 2018. Retrieved ProQuest Ebook Central, from https://ebookcentral.proquest.com/lib/nhsscotland-ebooks/detail.action?docID=5516881

3 Potential Impact of Maternal Obesity on the Child

Introduction

The previous chapter explored the potential impact of maternal obesity on the mother's health and, to some extent, the developing baby's during pregnancy. This chapter explores and discusses how maternal obesity can impact the child's health during pregnancy, labour and birth and throughout the lifelong continuum.

Discussing the potential consequences of maternal obesity on the developing child will undoubtedly be anxiety-provoking for professionals; however, practitioners have a responsibility to be truthful and provide women and families correct and accurate evidence-based information (Nursing and Midwifery Council [NMC] 2018) so that they might consider their lifestyle choices and, where appropriate, make 'positive changes' that may improve their own health and that of their unborn babies.

It is fundamental that, in addition to understanding the potential consequences of maternal obesity on the mother and baby's health, professionals have a clear understanding about the microbiological and physiological processes that occur during very early foetal and placental development that can predispose the child to sub-optimal health. Understanding these processes is a fundamental 'building block' that will underpin any information given to expectant parents about their current weight and lifestyle choices.

Early Life Programming

Maternal obesity and overnutrition are now well recognised risks for 'early life programming' (O'Reilly & Reynolds 2013), a phrase that describes how the developing foetus adapts to a 'toxic' environment. More scientifically, this means that their physiology has adapted for survival. Biochemical and physiological changes occur during phases of rapid cell growth in early pregnancy and are thought to be responsible for altered gene expression where a mother is obese (meaning that gene activity is altered from the normal) (Lean & Combet 2017). Recent findings suggest that this early life programming may have an impact on body systems of the foetus and cause autoimmune damage to organs such as the pancreas, which could predispose the child to diabetes later in life. Early life programming may also play a part in predisposing children to asthma and neuropsychiatric disorders (Lean & Combet 2017; Langley-Evans 2022).

Recent evidence also suggests that during very early pregnancy there is altered gene expression in the placenta that can impact on its growth, development and function throughout pregnancy which in turn impacts on the developing foetus, potentially setting the child on a course of developing sub-optimal health throughout life (Langley-Evans 2022).

DOI: 10.4324/9781003332398-4

Adipokines such as leptin and adiponectin are secreted by the placenta and enter the foetal circulation; these compounds are now understood to influence the development of adipose tissue in the developing foetus (Langley-Evans 2022). Furthermore, raised leptin levels found in the developing placenta are known to negatively impact on brain development in the foetus (Jaramillo-Ospina et al. 2021; Langley-Evans 2022). These biochemical processes that have been observed during very early pregnancy can and do have far-reaching implications for the offspring throughout the lifelong continuum. The remainder of this chapter examines in more detail some of the more commonly seen complications for babies of obese mothers, both in childhood and throughout the lifelong continuum.

Macrosomia

As discussed above, early biochemical changes in the placenta where a woman lives with an unhealthy weight can influence the amount of adipose tissue that is deposited in the developing baby. This can lead to the baby's becoming ***macrosomic***, a term used to describe foetal weight that is suspected of being greater than a specified threshold (Silasi 2018). In the UK, a baby is said to be macrosomic if it weighs 4.5 kg or more (Denison et al. 2018). The term macrosomia should not be confused with the expression 'large for gestation age' (LGA), which refers to babies that have grown above the 90th percentile for gestational age (Silasi 2018) but are still considered to be of 'normal' weight for gestational age.

The risk of injury to macrosomic babies is between 6 and 20 greater than that of normal-sized infants, and the typical injuries they may sustain are brachial plexus injury and fractures of the arm and/or shoulder as a result of shoulder dystocia. These babies may be more likely to require active resuscitation, and there is also a risk of their suffering from hypoglycaemia, polycythaemia and electrolyte disorders in the first few days of extra-uterine life (Silasi 2018; Beta et al. 2019). Depending upon the severity of injury, they may require admission to a neonatal unit (NNU) and risk separation from parents, which brings with it fears and anxieties for parents (Caporali et al. 2020; Adama et al. 2021).

Cerebral Palsy

This is an umbrella term that is used to describe many disturbances of motor function caused by injury to the foetal brain or neonatal brain (Zhang et al. 2018). In their meta-analysis, Zhang et al. (2018) found that the risk of cerebral palsy (CP) increased with maternal obesity levels. The physiological reasons for this are unknown; however, one must be cognisant that women who live with a raised body mass index (BMI) of at least 30 kg/m^2 are at risk of experiencing more complex labour and births, such as disordered labour, shoulder dystocia, operative delivery by obstetric forceps or Caesarean section, and that these circumstances may result in the baby's becoming hypoxic, which puts the child at risk of developing a brain injury and subsequent CP. Thus, the complex nature of labour and birth that some obese women experience, rather than maternal obesity itself, is likely to be the cause of hypoxia and CP.

Foetal Abnormality

Maternal obesity has been identified as a risk factor for foetal abnormalities such as cardiac defects, abnormalities of the nervous system, limb defects, orofacial cleft defects, and diaphragmatic hernia, and omphalocele (exomphalos) is amongst the most common (Persson et al. 2017). Rates of such abnormalities arising is increased depending upon level of obesity, and compared with their normal-weight counterparts, women who live with an unhealthy weight have a three-fold increased risk that their babies will be born with abnormalities (Persson et al. 2017; Denison et al. 2018).

Owing to excessive fat tissue in the maternal abdomen, it can be challenging to identify foetal abnormalities during ultrasound scanning. This is likely due to the physical distance between the abdominal wall and the foetus being increased, which in turn causes a reduction in the penetration of ultrasound waves reaching the foetus. To achieve good-quality images, the scan can take longer to perform than on a normal-weight woman, cause discomfort for her as well as potentially causing operator fatigue, which may also compromise the quality of images seen (Chodankar et al. 2018). These factors may increase the risk of any abnormalities in the foetus being 'missed' and result in families not receiving appropriate counselling about their abnormal foetus. It may also lead to delayed treatment being provided for such infants after birth which may impact upon the child's future quality of life. As discussed in the previous chapter, pregnancies of women who live with unhealthy weights are more likely to end in either miscarriage or stillbirth, and it is likely that undiagnosed foetal abnormalities will be the primary cause for some of these pregnancy losses occurring.

Women and their families have the right to be informed about how living with obesity can impact upon the baby and how and why some foetal abnormalities might be 'missed'.

Preterm Birth

Maternal obesity has been identified as an independent risk factor for preterm birth (Cnattingius et al. 2013; Sobczyk et al. 2022). In some cases, this is likely to be as a result of medical intervention due to diseases such as hypertension, pre-eclampsia and eclampsia or to diabetes becoming uncontrollable and necessitating delivery of the baby (Langley-Evans 2022). However, Liu et al. (2022) found that living with obesity was associated with higher incidences of spontaneous preterm labour and birth and premature rupture of the membranes (pre-labour) compared with women of normal weight; the reasons for this, however, are not clear, but as with disordered labour discussed earlier, the altered hormonal pathways may be affected and cause spontaneous labour to occur.

Preterm birth is associated with adverse outcomes for a neonate, such as infant mortality and morbidity, and long-term disabilities such as respiratory distress, chronic lung disease, apnoea, anaemia, patent ductus arteriosus, and proneness to infection due to having an immature immune system (Cnattingius et al. 2013; Petty 2017). When babies are admitted to the NNU, they are, out of necessity, separated from their parents, interrupting the normal flow of infant–parent bonding, particularly if the baby remains in the care of the NNU for several days, weeks or months. Admission to the NNU and subsequent separation have been found to lead to significant trauma symptoms for parents who have a preterm infant, and they have been found to develop alcohol use, depression, anxiety and stress within the first two weeks of the baby's admission (Dickson et al. 2022).

Petty (2017) asserts that the ideal situation would be to prevent preterm birth from occurring. Whilst no-one can predict how any pregnancy will end, it is important that women and their families be counselled about the risks of giving birth to a preterm infant when they live with an unhealthy weight and be given appropriate advice that might prevent such adversities. This is especially important when one considers the potential sequelae for parents if their babies are admitted to a NNU or neonatal intensive care unit (NICU) for prolonged periods. At such a time, it could be argued, parents need to maintain good health to support their sick baby.

Nutritional Challenges for the Baby

As discussed in the previous chapter, obese women are at increased risk of experiencing delayed lactogenesis and poor milk supply, putting the baby at risk of receiving formula supplementation with its incumbent risks of never establishing breastfeeding and being formula-fed. The risks of formula-feeding a baby are well understood; formula-fed babies are twice as likely to develop ear, gastro-intestinal or urinary tract infections, wheeze or eczema and juvenile diabetes (Petty 2017); in addition, preterm babies who are formula-fed are at greater risk of developing necrotizing enterocolitis (a potentially life-threatening condition) than their term counterparts (Petty 2017).

The United Nations International Children's Emergency Fund (UNICEF) (n.d.) recommends that all babies should be introduced to breastfeeding within the first hour of life and be exclusively breastfed for the first 6 months of life in order to reduce the risk of infections and to sustain optimal nutrition. Bentley et al. (2017) assert that obese women may need additional support if they are to successfully breastfeed. Supporting all women to breastfeed is one of the fundamental roles of the midwife; however, appropriate counselling about the potential difficulties that obese women may face when initiating breastfeeding may be of benefit so that women are forewarned about the potential challenges they may face when establishing early breastfeeding. Offering additional breastfeeding support soon after birth is likely to be necessary to ensure that this is a satisfying experience for mothers and offers optimal nutrition for their babies.

Long-Term Implications for Offspring

Whilst it is perhaps easy to understand that maternal overweight or obesity may impact upon a developing baby during pregnancy, it is now understood that there are long-term consequences for the children of obese adults (O'Reilly & Reynolds 2013; Reynolds et al. 2013; Langley-Evans et al. 2022) and these include, obesity, diabetes, neuropsychiatric disorders in childhood and early adulthood, and cardiac disease in later life (O'Reilly & Reynolds 2013; Reynolds et al. 2013; Langley-Evans et al. 2022).

Childhood Obesity

It is now understood that babies who are born to obese mothers are at risk of developing childhood and ongoing adult obesity. Previously, there may have been a tacit understanding that 'nurture' may have been responsible for this because children shared an obesogenic diet and lifestyle with their parents; there is now physiological evidence, however, to suggest that other factors influence this development (Langley-Evans 2022). Langley-Evans, (2022) found that children born to women who maintained their weight engaged in physical activity and who chose not to smoke during pregnancy were less likely to develop obesity at age 9–14 than those born to women who did not make these lifestyle changes. Similarly, Ounjaijean et al. (2021) found that young adults (19 to 22 years of age) who were born to obese women were at risk of obesity; that risk increased for every 1 kg/m^2 increase in the maternal BMI.

Living with increased risks of adiposity brings with it health risks for ongoing adulthood, meaning that the cycle of obesity is perpetuated. In addition, Ounjaijean et al. (2021) and Langley-Evans (2022) note that children born to obese mothers are at increased risk of developing metabolic syndrome in childhood, demonstrating that poor childhood health is perpetuated.

Metabolic Dysfunction in Children

Metabolic syndrome, as discussed in the previous chapter, is often seen in individuals who live with unhealthy weights and can include elements such as hypertension, obesity and glucose intolerance (Kaur 2014; Ellulu et al. 2016). However, maternal obesity is not just a risk factor for the *mother's* potential to develop metabolic syndrome; offspring of obese mothers are also at risk of developing metabolic syndrome as early as the age of 11 (Boney et al. 2005). This brings with it the risk of sub-optimal health throughout life.

Development of Diabetes During the Lifelong Continuum

The development of either type 1 (T1) or type 2 diabetes mellitus (T2DM) during the lifelong continuum is now a recognised risk for the child if that child is born to an obese woman (Ijäs et al. 2013; Langley-Evans 2022). This association was noted as long ago as 2008 during the Hyperglycaemia and Adverse Pregnancy Outcome (HAPO) study (Metzger et al. 2009). Langley-Evans (2022) explains that exposure to maternal obesity during pregnancy and the adverse uterine environment that a baby develops in may adversely impact upon specialist cell development in the foetal pancreas and cause remodelling of the organ itself. He concludes that these changes during foetal life increase the likelihood of children developing diabetes in childhood, adolescence or later life (Langley-Evans 2022).

This is of concern because diabetes is a chronic disease that requires significant medical supervision and brings with it ongoing long-term health risks. Caring for and helping young children to understand their disease and how to manage it will undoubtedly bring challenges for families and likely cause continued concern and anxiety about their children's long-term wellbeing. That is not to say that all children of obese mothers will go on to develop this disease, but professionals need to be cognisant of the potential risk in order to answer any questions accurately in the course of a consultation episode with expectant parents.

Childhood Neuropsychiatric Disorders

There is now a clear correlation between maternal obesity/overnutrition and the rate of neuropsychiatric conditions in offspring (Mina et al. 2017). These conditions include autism spectrum disorders, schizophrenic type behaviours and conditions such as attention-deficit/hyperactivity disorder (ADHD). Neuhaus et al. (2020) found that maternal overnutrition was an independent factor for these long-term conditions that will inevitably impact upon the individual's future quality of life.

The absolute mechanisms for children developing such disorders when born to obese mothers are not clear; however, Sullivan et al. (2015) suggest that, during pregnancy, the foetus is exposed to high levels of nutrients and endocrine compounds such as glucose, fatty acids, triglycerides, cytokines and, as mentioned previously, leptin. As a result of high glucose levels in the foetus, the foetal pancreas produces high levels of insulin; this is a normal physiological response. However, insulin plays an important role in foetal brain development (Simerly 2008), and hyperinsulinaemia during pregnancy may be responsible for altering early brain development and may be the cause of behavioural changes seen in older children (Sullivan et al. 2015).

In addition to hyperinsulinaemia, other compounds are thought to play roles in the development of these neuropsychiatric conditions. Leptin, an endocrine compound, is also thought to play a part in controlling stress and anxiety (Sullivan et al. 2015). Where a mother is obese, the foetus is exposed to high leptin levels and this overexposure to may alter mood and lead to behaviour changes in childhood and beyond (Sullivan et al. 2015). Additional complex pathways such as overexposure to cytokines, serotonin and dopamine may also have a role in causing these diseases to develop; however, currently, these theories have been arrived at using animal models.

Asthma

Asthma is an umbrella term used to describe a series of symptoms such as wheeze, chest tightness, breathlessness and unprovoked cough (Bush & Sonnappa 2020).

Asthmatic symptoms can become chronic and adversely affect a child's quality of life; both sub-optimal health and a poorer quality of life than their non-asthmatic peers can result in their being unable to take part in activities and missing days from school.

Although the biochemical and physiological mechanisms that may later predispose a developing foetus to asthma in childhood are not clear, an association between maternal obesity and childhood asthma has now been established (Patel et al. 2012; Polinski et al. 2017), and professionals need to be cognisant about this potential disease when counselling parents.

Conclusion

Children born to obese mothers are at risk of developing health problems not only during pregnancy and birth but throughout the lifelong continuum. Discerning the right time for individuals to discuss these risks will not be an easy task and will rely on professionals developing the trusting relationship that is strived for in midwifery practice (NMC 2019). However, in some cases, holding these difficult conversations and supporting families to make lifestyle choices may promote good health for the child in the long term. Despite this, it is likely that, for some parents, being informed about these potential risks will be anxiety-provoking, just as to deliver such messages may be anxiety-provoking for professionals. This brings us back to the need to develop skills in constructing effective consultation episodes that allow honest information exchange with parents and provide space for emotions to be released.

The body of scientific evidence is growing with respect to the health risks that children born to obese mothers might face and cannot be ignored. Professionals therefore have a responsibility to provide accurate and evidence-based information about potential birth complications and the risks they pose to the baby during pregnancy, the neonatal period and throughout the lifelong continuum. Holding such discussions, however, is likely to be anxiety-provoking for professionals, especially if they have no further information to provide with respect to promoting and protecting future health. However, there is evidence available to suggest that improving diet and exercise can protect both the mother and baby's health during pregnancy and lead to optimal pregnancy outcomes.

Having informed families about the potential risks of living with an unhealthy weight during pregnancy, professionals need to be knowledgeable about the measures one can take with respect to protecting and promoting good health and be able to provide good advice and support to families.

The next few chapters discuss the lifestyle measures that can improve health outcomes for mothers, babies and families. Please now take time to consider the questions posed in Box 3.1.

Box 3.1 Professional Reflective Questions

- Reflect upon some of your experiences in clinical practice and consider the following questions and statements.
  - Did you encounter any families who were advised that a foetus may have an abnormality but the diagnosis was uncertain because of maternal obesity?
  - If so, was there any further discussion with the midwife and/or obstetrician as to why this was necessary?
  - If there was further discussion, did you consider that it was dealt with effectively where the topic of maternal obesity wasn't shied away from?
  - Now consider how you might construct a discussion with a family that may be expecting a baby with an abnormality.
    - What language might you use?
    - How might you explain that obesity may have played a part in obscuring the view of the baby's structures at scan?
    - What resources might you signpost such families to?
- Now consider some consultations that you have witnessed that have been undertaken by medical staff with respect to potential foetal abnormality.
  - How did the medical staff initiate the conversation?
  - In your opinion, was this done in an effective manner that allowed for honest exchange between the clinician and the parents?
  - Was the model of consultation you witnessed one that you would like to develop in your own professional repertoire?
- Consider some postnatal scenarios that you may have witnessed or been involved in where the mother lived with obesity.
  - Were there many incidences where the baby suffered a complication during birth?
  - Was there any indication that the mother was made aware that her unhealthy weight may have been a contributing factor for sub-optimal health in the baby?
  - Did any professionals raise the issue with the mother and provide any lifestyle guidance about protecting future health?

Consider how, during your consultation episodes, you might incorporate discussion about the baby's health with women and their families when they live with an unhealthy weight.

References

Adama, E. A., Adula, E, Baye, S., & Morellius, S. (2021). Support needs of parents in neonatal intensive care: An integrative review. *Journal of Clinical Nursing*. https://doi.org/10.1111nity/jocn.15972

Bentley, J. P., Nassar, N., Porter, M., Vroome, M., Yip, E., & Ampt, A. J. (2017). Formula supplementation in hospital and subsequent feeding at discharge among women who intended to exclusively breastfeed: An administrative data retrospective cohort study. *Birth (Berkeley, Calif.)*, *44*(4), 352–362. https://doi.org/10.1111/birt.12300

Beta, J., Khan, N., Khalil, A., Fiolna, M., Ramadan, G., & Akolekar, R. (2019). Maternal and neonatal complications of fetal macrosomia: Systematic review and meta-analysis. *Ultrasound in Obstetrics & Gynecology*, *54*(3), 308–318. https://doi.org/10.1002/uog.20279

Boney, C. M., Verma, A., Tucker, R., & Vohr, B. R. (2005). Metabolic syndrome in childhood: Association with birth weight, maternal obesity, and gestational diabetes mellitus. *Pediatrics*, *115*(3), e290–e296. https://doi.org/10.1542/peds.2004-1808

Bush, A., & Sonnappa, S. (2020). Confirming the diagnosis of severe asthma in children. In E. Forno & S. Saglani (Eds.), *Severe asthma in children and adolescents* (pp. 49–71). Springer. https://doi.org/10.1007/978-3-030-27431-3_3

Caporali, C., Pisoni, C., Gasparini, L., Ballante, E., Zecca, M., Orcesi, S., & Provenzi, L. (2020). A global perspective on parental stress in the neonatal intensive care unit: A meta-analytic study. *Journal of Perinatology*, *40*(12), 1739–1752. https://doi.org/10.1038/s41372-020-00798-6

Chodankar, R., Middleton, G., Lim, C., & Mahmood, T. (2018). Obesity in pregnancy. *Obstetrics, Gynaecology and Reproductive Medicine*, *28*(2), 53–56. https://doi.org/10.1016/j.ogrm.2017.11.003

Cnattingius S., Villamor E., Johansson S., et al. (2013). Maternal obesity and risk of preterm delivery. *JAMA*, 309(22), 2362–2370. https://doi.org/10.1001/jama.2013.6295

Crofts, J., Draycott, T., Montague, I., Winter, C., & Fox, R. (2012). *Shoulder Dystocia*. Retrieved November 23, 2023, from https://www.rcog.org.uk/guidance/browse-all-guidance/green-top-guidelines/shoulder-dystocia-green-top-guideline-no-42/

Denison, F. C., Aedla, N. R., Keag, O., Hor, K., Reynolds, R. M., Milne, A., Diamond, A., Amir, L., Bodnar, L. M., Beckett, V., Bouch, C., Cousins, J., Duckitt, K., Fox, K. A., Fraser, D., McCurdy, R. J., Salama, H., Salama, H. S., Smith, G. C. S., ... Thomson, A. J. (2018). Care of women with obesity in pregnancy green-top guideline no. 72. *BJOG: An International Journal of Obstetrics and Gynaecology*, *126*(3), E62–E106. https://doi.org/10.1111/1471-0528.15386

Dickinson, C., Vangaveti, V.N., & Browne, A. (2022). Psychological impact of neonatal intensive care unit admissions on parents: A regional perspective. *The Australian Journal of Rural Health*, https://doi.org/10.1111/ajr.12841

Ellulu, M. S., Patimah, I., Khaza'ai, H., Rahmat, A., & Abed, Y. (2016). Obesity and inflammation: the linking mechanism and the complications. *Archives of Medical Science*, *13*(4), 851–863. https://doi.org/10.5114%2Faoms.2016.58928

Ijäs, H., Morin-Papunen, L., Keränen, A. K., Bloigu, R., Ruokonen, A., Puukka, K., Ebeling, T., Raudaskoski, T., & Vääräsmäki, M. (2013). Pre-pregnancy overweight overtakes gestational diabetes as a risk factor for subsequent metabolic syndrome. *European Journal of Endocrinology*, *169*(5), 605–611. https://doi.org/10.1530/EJE-13-0412

Jaramillo-Ospina, Á., Castaño-Moreno, E., Muñoz-Muñoz, E., Krause, B. J., Uauy, R., Casanello, P., & Castro-Rodriguez, J. A. (August 2021). Maternal obesity is associated with higher cord blood adipokines in offspring most notably in females. *Journal of Pediatric Gastroenterology and Nutrition*, *73*(2), 264–270. https://doi.org/10.1097/mpg.0000000000003172

Kaur, J. (2014). A comprehensive review on metabolic syndrome. *Cardiology and Research Practice*. https://doi.org/10.1155/2014/943162

Langley-Evans S. C. (2022). Early life programming of health and disease: The long-term consequences of obesity in pregnancy. *Journal of Human Nutrition and Dietetics: The Official Journal of the British Dietetic Association*, *35*(5), 816–832. https://doi.org/10.1111/jhn.13023

Langley-Evans, S. C., Pearce, J., & Ellis, S. (2022). Overweight, obesity and excessive weight gain in pregnancy as risk factors for adverse pregnancy outcomes: A narrative review. *Journal of Human Nutrition and Dietetics*, *35*(2), 250–264. https://doi.org/10.1111/jhn.12999

Lean, M., & Combet, E. (2017). *Barasi's Human Nutrition, A health perspective* (3rd ed.). CRC Press.

Liu, K., Chen, Y., Tong, J., Yin, A., Wu, L., & Niu, J. (2022). Association of maternal obesity with preterm birth phenotype and mediation effects of gestational diabetes mellitus and preeclampsia: A prospective cohort study. *BMC Pregnancy and Childbirth*, *22*(1), 1–9. https://doi.org/10.1186/s12884-022-04780-2

Metzger, B. E., Lowe, L. P., Dyer, A. R., Trimble, E. R., Sheridan, B., Hod, M., Chen, R., Yogev, Y., Coustan, D. R., Catalano, P. M., Giles, W., Lowe, J., Hadden, D. R., Persson, B., & Oats, J. J. N. (2009). Hyperglycemia and adverse pregnancy outcome (HAPO) study associations with neonatal anthropometrics. *Diabetes (New York, N.Y.)*, *58*(2), 453–459. https://doi.org/10.2337/db08-1112

Mina, T. H., Lahti, M., Drake, A. J., Räikkönen, K., Minnis, H., Denison, F. C., Norman, J. E., & Reynolds, R. M. (2017). Prenatal exposure to very severe maternal obesity is associated with adverse neuropsychiatric outcomes in children. *Psychological Medicine*, *47*(2), 353–362. https://doi.org/10.1017/S0033291716002452

Neuhaus, Z. F., Gutvirtz, G., Pariente, G., Wainstock, T., Landau, D., & Sheiner, E. (2020). Maternal obesity and long-term neuropsychiatric morbidity of the offspring. *Archives of Gynecology and Obstetrics*, *301*(1), 143–149. https://doi.org/10.1007/s00404-020-05432-6

Nursing and Midwifery Council. (2018). *The Code*. Retrieved November 23, 2023, from https://www.nmc.org.uk/standards/code/

Nursing and Midwifery Council. (2019). Standards of Proficiency for Midwives. Retrieved November 23, 2023, from https://www.nmc.org.uk/standards/midwifery/education

O'Reilly, J. R., & Reynolds, R. M. (2013). The risk of maternal obesity to the long-term health of the offspring. *Clinical Endocrinology (Oxford)*, *78*(1), 9–16. https://doi.org/10.1111/cen.12055

Ounjaijean, S., Wongthanee, A., Kulprachakarn, K., Rerkasem, A., Pruenglampoo, S., Mangklabruks, A., Rerkasem, K., & Derraik, J. G. B. (2021). Higher maternal BMI early in pregnancy is associated with overweight and obesity in young adult offspring in Thailand. *BMC Public Health*, *21*(1), 724–724. https://doi.org/10.1186/s12889-021-10678-z

Patel, S. P., Rodriguez, A., Little, M. P., Elliott, P., Pekkanen, J., Hartikainen, A.-L., Pouta, A., Laitinen, J., Harju, T., Canoy, D., & Järvelin, M.-R. (2012). Associations between pre-pregnancy obesity and asthma symptoms in adolescents. *Journal of Epidemiology and Community Health (1979)*, *66*(9), 809–814. https://doi.org/10.1136/jech.2011.133777

Persson, C. S., Villamor, E., Söderling, J., Pasternak, B., Stephansson, O., & Neovius, M. (2017). Risk of major congenital malformations in relation to maternal overweight and obesity severity: cohort study of 1.2 million singletons. *BMJ*, *357*(8110), j2563–j2563. https://doi.org/10.1136/bmj.j2563

Petty, J. (2017). The preterm baby and the small baby. In S. Macdonald & G. Johnson (Eds.), *Mayes' midwifery* (15th ed., pp. 790–808). Elsevier.

Polinski, K. J., Liu, J., Boghossian, N. S., & McLain, A. C. (2017). Maternal obesity, gestational weight gain, and asthma in offspring. *Preventing Chronic Disease*, *14*, E109. https://doi.org/10.5888/pcd14.170196

Reynolds, R. M., Allan, K. M., Raja, E. A., Battacharya, S., McNeill, G., Hannaford, P. C., Sarwar, N., Lee, A. J., Bhattacharya, S., & Norman, J. E. (2013). Maternal obesity during pregnancy and premature mortality from cardiovascular event in adult offspring: Follow-up of 1 323 275 person years. *BMJ Open*, 10. https://doi.org/10.1136/bmj.f4539

Silasi, M. (2018). Fetal macrosomia. In. J. A. Copel (Ed.), *Obstetric imaging: Fetal diagnosis and care* (2nd ed., pp. 460–462). Elsevier. https://doi.org/10.1016/C2014-0-00100-1

Simerly, R. B. (2008). Hypothalamic substrates of metabolic imprinting. *Physiology & Behavior*, *94*(1), 79–89. https://doi.org/10.1016/j.physbeh.2007.11.023

Sobczyk, K., Holecki, T., Woźniak-Holecka, J., & Grajek, M. (2022). Does maternal obesity affect preterm birth? Documentary cohort study of preterm in firstborns-silesia (Poland). *Children (Basel, Switzerland)*, *9*(7), 1007. https://doi.org/10.3390/children9071007

Sullivan, E. L., Riper, K. M., Lockard, R., & Valleau, J. C. (2015). Maternal high-fat diet programming of the neuroendocrine system and behavior. *Hormones and Behavior*, *76*, 153–161. https://doi.org/10.1016/j.yhbeh.2015.04.008

UNICEF. (n.d.). The Baby Friendly Initiative. Retrieved 23 November 2023, from, https://www.unicef.org.uk/babyfriendly/

Zhang, J., Peng, L., Chang, Q., Xu, R., Zhong, N., Huang, Q., Zhong, M., & Yu, Y. (2018). Maternal obesity and risk of cerebral palsy in children: A systematic review and meta-analysis. *Developmental Medicine and Child Neurology*, *61*(1), 31–38. https://doi.org/10.1111/dmcn.13982

4 Weight Gain, Diet, Nutrition and Eating during Pregnancy

Introduction

The previous two chapters have focused on the potential risks of living with an unhealthy weight to both women and their unborn babies. The thought of discussing some of the potentially serious issues that women and babies may encounter may cause anxiety for students and newly registered professionals. However, this chapter is rather more positive; it focuses on optimising nutritional intake and on weight *maintenance* and *stabilisation* and discusses some of the evidence around this approach. There is some discussion with respect to optimal weight gain during pregnancy.

Optimal nutrition is discussed, and there is guidance for professionals as to what advice obese women should be receiving with respect to diet and nutritional intake. Eating and socialising are meshed in society, and this is acknowledged and explored in this chapter.

Calorific Needs

A calorie is a measurement of energy. It is the amount of energy that is required to heat 1 ml of water by 1° Celsius (Lean & Combet 2017), and the basic calorific requirements for a typical woman are as follows:

- Breakfast: 300–500 kcal
- Lunch: 500–700 kcal
- Dinner: 500–700 kcal
- Two additional snacks of 150 kcal each

(Lean & Combet 2017, p. 13)

The calorific needs during pregnancy are similar to those required for women who are not pregnant – except during the third trimester, when there is an increased need of about 200 kcal/day. However, people eat food as food and not as calories or nutrients, so professionals will need to be in possession of appropriate evidence-based knowledge with respect to the nutritional value of commonly chosen foods if they are to advise and guide women in their food choices appropriately.

Optimal Weight Gain in Pregnancy

In 2009, the USA Institute of Medicine (ACOG 2009) suggested that gestational weight gain (GWG) should be proportionate to the baseline body mass index (BMI) level (see Table 4.1 for detail), and it is this guide that is often used in practice. However, these

DOI: 10.4324/9781003332398-5

Table 4.1 Recommended weight gain during pregnancy according to baseline body mass index (BMI)

Baseline BMI prior to pregnancy	*Recommended weight gain*
BMI <18.5 kg/m^2	12.4–17.9 kg
BMI 18.5–24.9 kg/m^2 (normal weight)	11.5–15.8 kg
BMI 25.1–29.9 kg/m^2 (overweight)	7–11.5 kg
BMI >30 kg/m^2 (obese)	5–9 kg

Source: Adapted from the USA Institute of Medicine (2009).

recommendations have been based on observational studies that considered the prevention of 'large for gestational age' and 'small for gestational age' babies and the reduction in numbers of Caesarean sections rather than on findings from randomised controlled trials (RCTs) (Denison et al. 2018). Furthermore, there is limited evidence about the effects of GWG during pregnancy and how the particular gestation at which it occurs impacts on the health of mother and baby. Findings from a systematic review (Faucher & Barger 2015) suggest that a more detailed approach may be advantageous and that weight gain recommendations during pregnancy should be adjusted depending upon the category of obesity with which someone lives rather than just upon the BMI measurement being over 30 kg/m^2. However, it is understood that excessive GWG can impact negatively on a woman or baby's health antenatally and beyond pregnancy.

Denison et al. (2018) acknowledge the lack of evidence with respect to optimal GWG and suggest that women should be advised to focus on a 'healthy diet' rather than on weight targets. Owing to its association with babies being born that are small for gestation age (SGA), deliberate weight loss by restricting calories during pregnancy is not recommended (Lean & Combet 2017; Denison et al. 2018). In some cases, however, women may lose weight during pregnancy because of complications such as hyperemesis gravidarum or other gastro-intestinal problems. Specialist advice from dietetic services should be sought if this eventuality occurs. It is also worth noting that women who increase the quality of their diets and engage in physical activity may also experience incidental weight loss; in such cases, foetal growth should be closely observed and ultrasound scan for foetal growth estimation ordered. Obstetric and dietetic review may also be appropriate.

What Is Meant by 'Healthy Diet'?

The term 'a healthy and balanced diet' is often heard in healthcare contexts; however, what this means is likely to differ between individuals. Lean and Combet (2017) explain that there is not a generic definition of what 'healthy' actually means and argue that it is a term used for marketing foods that will result in weight loss. This is not helpful for professionals who are striving to provide accurate information for all pregnant women as well as women who live with unhealthy weights. Therefore, if they are to guide and support women to make dietary changes and optimise their health and pregnancy outcomes, professionals who provide maternity care need to be equipped with accurate knowledge about what nutritionally optimal foods are.

One of the challenges that professionals face with respect to providing nutritional advice is to consider that individuals will have varying food preferences. Therefore, as discussed in Chapter 1, professionals will need to explore the individual's current dietary habits and preferences and offer advice on how to optimise it where appropriate. When an obese woman's diet is being assessed, this again may prove challenging because evidence has shown that obese people commonly under-report their calorific intake (Lean & Combet 2017). In order to support women, professionals therefore will have to construct a consultation episode that is meaningful and include within it topics that are relevant to that particular woman and her social context.

With respect to diet, obese women should be given accurate advice that focuses on three principles: increasing the intake of fruit and vegetables, decreasing consumption of food with high glycaemic indices and observing portion control (Lean & Combet 2017; Denison et al. 2018). This approach aims to stabilise weight and not reduce it whilst ensuring that the woman receives adequate intake of nutrients to maintain good health for her and her developing baby.

The focus should be not to restrict or 'ban' any food but to advise women to be mindful about the foods that they do choose and to ensure that there is balance of all foods and therefore nutrients in their diets. A nutritionally optimal diet needs to consist of proteins, vitamins and minerals and carbohydrates; a balance of these compounds will ensure that the body receives enough energy for cell division and repair and normal body functioning. A summary of the foods that contain these nutrients can be seen in Table 4.2 and Table 4.3 provides an overview of how nutrients are used in the body.

Limiting Weight Gain in Pregnancy

There have been significant RCTs conducted in the UK (McGiveron et al. 2015; Flynn et al. 2016), Australia (Dodd et al. 2016) and Sweden (Haby et al. 2015) aimed at exploring whether additional sessions with appropriately educated professionals offering advice about diet and lifestyle were effective in optimising health and reducing the incidence of poor pregnancy outcomes. In all four studies, women were randomly assigned either to an intervention group where diet and lifestyle advice was given or to a 'standard care' group that provided routine care only. The results in all four studies demonstrated that providing additional lifestyle advice to women was not harmful and that women appreciated the information given, and McGiveron et al. (2015) found that limiting weigh gain also resulted in a reduction of hypertension disorders. Of note, Flynn et al. (2016) concluded that providing advice with respect to diet and lifestyle during antenatal appointments was an approach that could be further explored and used during routine antenatal care.

Langley-Evans and Ellis (2022) make an interesting point by saying that, in the UK, providing advice with respect to weight management during pregnancy is a missed opportunity. Denison et al. (2018) suggest that women should be advised about the benefits of optimising their weight prior to conception and the benefits of losing additional weight after they have finished breastfeeding. During pregnancy however, women should be advised to stabilise their weight and focus on a nutritionally optimal diet. Currently during pregnancy (in the UK), maternal weight is somewhat ignored and routine weighing to assess GWG is not done. This may be due to confusion amongst professionals as to what the optimal weight gain should be (as discussed earlier) or it may be that a 'tick box' on institutional questionnaires does not prompt professionals to undertake routine weighing (Greig et al. 2021).

Not providing information about the risks of living with obesity during pregnancy to women and their families is no longer an option. Women have the right to be informed

Table 4.2 Summary of nutritionally optimal foods

Foods/food groups	*Nutritional compounds*	*Function in the body*
Meats, poultry, fish, cheese, milk, eggs, beans, peas, pulses, corn and wheat products, yeast and soya	Proteins and amino acids	Cell development, antibody development Regulation of acid–base balance Transport of free fatty acids and lipids
Fish, animal fats, olive oil, nuts and avocado	Essential fatty acids	Energy and heat insulation A carrier for fat-soluble vitamins
Potatoes, bread, cereals, pasta, rice and intrinsic sugars found in fruit and vegetables. Extrinsic sugars found in fruit juice, jams, cakes and biscuits	Carbohydrates	These are easily digested nutrients that are stored as glycogen in the liver. Carbohydrate intake should equate to about half of all food consumed (Jewell 2017, p. 263)
Fish oils, eggs and dairy produce Apricots, carrots and other orange/yellow vegetables Green leafy vegetables	Vitamins (A–E) and minerals	Cell growth and repair Efficient immune system Synthesis of ribonucleic acid (RNA) Protein metabolism Detoxifying agent Antioxidant
Whole grain nuts, leafy green vegetables, oranges, broccoli, tuna and liver (not recommended during pregnancy)	Folic acid	Production of erythrocytes Maintenance of the nervous system Gastro-intestinal tract functioning Leucocyte production Choline and methionine production Associated with low risk of neural tube disorders in the developing foetus
Fish, shellfish, liver, red meat, eggs, milk, nuts and wholegrains, mushrooms and leafy green vegetables	Zinc	Cell development and repair in the vital organs, including the brain Skeletal, skin and hair growth
Red meats, fish, eggs, wholemeal bread, cereals, potatoes, dried fruits and nuts, and pulses, including kidney beans, lentils and chickpeas.	Iron	Production of red blood cells and oxygenation of tissues Protein metabolism Bone growth Efficient immunity and disease resistance

Sources: Adapted from Lean and Combet 2017, Jewell 2017.

about the potential health risks of living with obesity whilst pregnant and to be guided and supported with respect to optimising their dietary and lifestyle choices.

Advice Giving (Diet)

Providing this basic advice sounds relatively simple, but when such information is being provided to an individual who is already obese, a more detailed approach is likely to be required. Individuals are overweight or obese because there is an energy imbalance: they have taken in more energy (calories) than they have expended (WHO 2021). A detailed exploration of both their dietary and their physical activity habits will be required so that appropriate constructive advice can be offered that suits the individual's needs and supports them in optimising their dietary habits and in turn their health.

Table 4.3 Overview of vitamins required for good health

Nutrient	*Function in the body*
Thiamin (vitamin B_1)	Maintains nerves Digestion of carbohydrates
Riboflavin (vitamin B_2)	Metabolism of fats and carbohydrates Efficient wound-healing Hormonal regulation
Niacin (vitamin B_3)	Metabolism of fats, proteins and carbohydrates Hormonal regulation Converts food to energy
Pyridoxine (vitamin B_6)	Antibiotic production Production of erythrocytes Synthesises proteins Maintenance of the nervous system Releases stored glycogen (in the liver)
Cobalamin (vitamin B_{12})	Erythrocyte production and efficient bone-marrow function RNA and DNA development Carbohydrate metabolism Regulation of blood acid levels
Vitamin C	Cell and bone health Wound healing Amino acid metabolism Has a role in iron absorption
Vitamin D	Calcium absorption Maintains bones and teeth Maintains renal, cardiac and nervous systems Plays a part in coagulation
Vitamin E	Maintains erythrocyte levels Sustains major body functions Retards aging Plays a part in stress responses

Sources: Adapted from Jewell 2017.

This in itself may be fraught with difficulty, particularly if the individual feels that they are being 'lectured' to and that their individual context is not being considered. Constructing a conversation that allows the individual to consider their diet and lifestyle habits for themselves and understand how they can make positive changes to their diet and lifestyle will need careful thought. Professionals need to give people time and space to consider this and acknowledge that it may be beneficial to schedule additional appointments to discuss diet and lifestyle that don't align with current antenatal routines in the UK.

Cooking Skills and Changing Family Structures

It is now accepted that many women work outside the home and are not the traditional family member to oversee grocery shopping and the cooking of meals. This has resulted in increased purchases of convenience foods and the loss of cooking skills; furthermore, family members now often choose individual times to eat (Lean & Combet 2017). These changes to family life may have impacted upon some pregnant women who are now presenting for maternity care, and it is likely that some of them will not have learned cooking skills in the home and may have been brought up eating convenience and processed foods. In recognition of these issues, the 'Let's Get Cooking' network was launched in the UK in 2007 by the British Dietetic Association (DBA) and was aimed at improving both diet literacy and cooking skills for children and parents alike. This consists of community spaces being used to educate parents and children about nutrition and families being involved in cookery classes, preparing food together. Results have shown that 70% of participants learned a new healthy eating skill, 50% of children intended to increase their intake of healthy foods and 87% of participants transferred and practised their skills at home (Carter 2010).

Signposting some women and their families to cookery clubs such as this may be beneficial (if they are locally available); however, as has been previously said, this depends on individual contexts and preferences and should be provided as a suggestion only. Being aware of local charitable organisations that can support families with respect to diet literacy and cooking skills is important because a healthcare professional cannot 'do it all,' and in tightly scheduled appointments, it is not reasonable to expect maternity professionals to discuss how to cook nutritionally valuable meals with families and calls into question the Scope of Practice (NMC 2018). Professionals also need to be cognisant that some families may have limited access to cooking facilities in the home.

Additional Considerations with Food Habits

Social Context and Cost-of-Living Crisis

At the time of writing this book, the UK was experiencing a cost-of-living crisis with families struggling to either pay energy bills or buy food. Such crises undoubtedly impact upon food choices, especially when one considers that foods high in fats, sugar and salts tend to be cheaper than those that are nutritionally more valuable (Lean & Combet 2017). Professionals therefore need to guide individuals' understanding about the foods that are affordable and of nutritional value. Fresh fruit and vegetables tend to be more expensive than tinned or frozen alternatives; however, using these alternatives can be an effective way of increasing fibre and vitamin intake while reducing intake of foods that are high in fat, sugar and salt.

Being in possession of evidence-based nutritional knowledge and exploring individuals' preferences and contexts will be key if conversations around dietary changes are to be constructed in a meaningful way that support women to make lifestyle changes. Another function of such conversations is to discern and assess women's baseline knowledge about nutritional literacy.

The Social Aspect of Food

Eating is not just a means of nourishing our bodies, it is associated with socialising. It is a pleasurable experience to enjoy food with family and friends either in the home or at celebratory events. In addition, pregnancy is often a time when women have time to socialise with new friends and families, often engaging in eating events. These occasions often result in additional calories being eaten, and often the food that is available is high in sugar, salt and fat. Despite these potential eating 'hazards', women should be advised to enjoy all social engagements but to be mindful of their food choices, choosing foods that are lower in sugar, salt and fat, and mindful about how much food they are consuming.

Snacks

Whilst eating many snacks that are high in sugar, salt and fat is often discouraged, for some additional calories between meals is beneficial. However, it is important that woman be informed that, during pregnancy, there is a need to increase calorie intake only during the last trimester of pregnancy and that only 150 kcal are required (Lean & Combet 2017). The DBA acknowledges that 'snacking' can have benefits such as improving the

Box 4.1 Personal Reflective Questions

- Prior to reading this chapter, explore your baseline knowledge about diet and nutrition.
  - Do you consider that you have been knowledgeable about the nutrients required for good health?
  - Consider where you acquired your knowledge surrounding nutrition. Was it from professional sources or general media?
- Consider how you will remain updated with respect to this aspect of care as your practice continues to develop.
  - Consider how much emphasis you have placed on educating women about nutrition previously and what will now influence your practice.
- Going forward, consider how confident you might be when raising the topic of a nutritionally rich diet with women.
  - How will you adapt and develop your consultation skills to include meaningful discussion around this topic as your practice develops?
  - What additional questions, if any, do you ask women about their particular food preferences and behaviours?
  - Consider how often you use the term 'healthy diet'. What term might you consider using in the future?
  - Having read this chapter, explain how your knowledge and confidence may have changed with respect to providing nutritional advice.
- Now that you have read this chapter and Chapter 1, consider how you might start to develop a meaningful conversation about eating a nutritionally valuable diet.
  - Consider how you will discern an individual's personal context with respect to their dietary choices.
  - What questions and statements might you use when informing people about the content of their appointment with you?
  - What questions or statements might you use when continuing a conversation about dietary choices?
- Consider how you will continue to remain current with this aspect of health.
  - What professional literature will you access going forward?
  - What literature will you signpost women to with respect to choosing nutritionally valuable foods?

Consider what other colleague you may approach to ask for advice with respect to giving personalised information to women with respect to diet.

nutritional intake and preventing overeating (if the chosen food has a low glycaemic index) at the next meal. Like all other foods, snacks come from the various food groups, and not all of them are considered 'unhealthy'; for example, fruit would be an optimal choice. However, this depends upon their socio-economic situation, and professionals need to be cognisant that not all women are in a position to choose more nutritionally valuable snacks. Women should therefore be advised to choose foods from any of the food groups, but if they choose food that is high in sugar, fats and salt, the advice should be to take smaller or 'fun size' portions. In addition, practical advice should be given with respect to keeping nutritionally optimal snacks on hand when they go about their daily business (BDA 2021). Now please consider the questions posed in Box 4.1.

References

American College of Obstetricians and Gynaecology. (2009) [reaffirmed 2023]. *Weight gain during pregnancy*. Retrieved from https://www.acog.org/clinical/clinical-guidance/committee-opinion/articles/2013/01/weight-gain-during-pregnancy

British Dietetic Association. (2021). *Snacking worries*. Retrieved from https://www.bda.uk.com/resource/healthy-snacks.html

Carter, W. (2010). Let's get cooking – A national network of healthy cooking clubs. *Nutrition Bulletin*, *35*(1), 57–59. https://doi.org/10.1111/j.1467-3010.2009.01804.x

Denison, F. C., Aedla, N. R., Keag, O., Hor, K., Reynolds, R. M., Milne, A., Diamond, A., Amir, L., Bodnar, L. M., Beckett, V., Bouch, C., Cousins, J., Duckitt, K., Fox, K. A., Fraser, D., McCurdy, R. J., Salama, H., Salama, H. S., Smith, G. C. S., ... Thomson, A. J. (2018). Care of women with obesity in pregnancy green-top guideline no. 72. *BJOG: An International Journal of Obstetrics and Gynaecology*, *126*(3), E62–E106. https://doi.org/10.1111/1471-0528.15386

Dodd, N. A., Moran, L. J., Deussen, A. R., Grivell, R. M., Yelland, L. N., Crowther, C. A., McPhee, A. J., Wittert, G., Owens, J. A., Turnbull, D., & Robinson, J. S. (2016). The effect of antenatal dietary and lifestyle advice for women who are overweight or obese on emotional well-being: The LIMIT randomized trial. *Acta Obstetricia et Gynecologica Scandinavica*, *95*(3), 309–318. https://doi.org/10.1111/aogs.12832

Faucher, M. A., & Barger, M. K. (2015). Gestational weight gain in obese women by class of obesity and select maternal/newborn outcomes: A systematic review. *Women and Birth: Journal of the Australian College of Midwives*, *28*(3), e70–e79. https://doi.org/10.1016/j.wombi.2015.03.006

Flynn, S. P. T., Patel, N., Barr, S., Bell, R., Briley, A. L., Godfrey, K. M., Nelson, S. M., Oteng-Ntim, E., Robinson, S. M., Sanders, T. A., Sattar, N., Wardle, J., Poston, L., & Goff, L. M. (2016). Dietary patterns in obese pregnant women; influence of a behavioral intervention of diet and physical activity in the UPBEAT randomized controlled trial. *The International Journal of Behavioral Nutrition and Physical Activity*, *13*(1), 124–124. https://doi.org/10.1186/s12966-016-0450-2

Greig, Y., Williams, A. F., & Coulter-Smith, M. (2021). Obesity matters: The skills that strengthen midwifery practice when caring for obese pregnant women. *British Journal of Midwifery*, *29*(5), 278–285. https://doi.org/10.12968/bjom.2021.29.5.278

Haby, G. A., Hanas, R., & Premberg, Å. (2015). Mighty Mums – An antenatal health care intervention can reduce gestational weight gain in women with obesity. *Midwifery*, *31*(7), 685–692. https://doi.org/10.1016/j.midw.2015.03.014

Jewell, K. (2017). Nutrition. In S. Macdonald & G. Johnson (Eds.), *Mayes' midwifery* (15th ed., pp. 262–287). Elsevier.

Langley-Evans, P. J., & Ellis, S. (2022). Overweight, obesity and excessive weight gain in pregnancy as risk factors for adverse pregnancy outcomes: A narrative review. *Journal of Human Nutrition and Dietetics*, *35*(2), 250–264. https://doi.org/10.1111/jhn.12999

Lean, M., & Combet, E. (2017). *Barasi's human nutrition, A health perspective* (3rd ed.). CRC Press.

McGiveron, F. S., Pearce, J., Taylor, M. A., McMullen, S., & Langley-Evans, S. C. (2015). Limiting antenatal weight gain improves maternal health outcomes in severely obese pregnant women: Findings of a pragmatic evaluation of a midwife-led intervention. *Journal of Human Nutrition and Dietetics*, *28*(s1), 29–37. https://doi.org/10.1111/jhn.12240

Nursing and Midwifery Council. (2018). *The Code*. Retrieved November 23, 2023, from https://www.nmc.org.uk/standards/code/

World Health Organisation. (2021). *Obesity and overweight*. Retrieved from https://www.who.int/news-room/fact-sheets/detail/obesity-and-overweight

5 Physical Activity

Introduction

This chapter discusses the definitions of physical activity, physical inactivity and sedentary behaviour according to the World Health Organization (WHO) (2022). It provides an overview of the physiological impact of being inactive and explains why engaging in physical activity at any level is beneficial for the health of individuals, the wider population and pregnant women. Some of the barriers and facilitators that exist for pregnant women with respect to exercise are discussed. Current UK physical activity guidance is discussed, and suggestions as to how midwives might inform women about increasing their daily activity are provided.

Physical Activity as Protector of Health

It is now understood that engaging in physical activity has significant health benefits for everyone and protects people from developing non-communicable diseases such as type 2 diabetes mellitus (T2DM), cardiovascular disease and mental health disorders (including dementia). High costs are associated with treating preventable illnesses, and this places a burden on governments in terms of healthcare provision and social planning (WHO 2022). Conversely, and not surprisingly, being inactive increases our risks of developing non-communicable diseases, and the term 'sedentary behaviours' is now being used by the WHO (2022) to describe what may be interpreted as conscious inactivity:

> Sedentary behaviour is defined as any waking behaviour characterized by an energy expenditure ≤1.5 metabolic equivalents, such as sitting, reclining or lying down.
>
> (WHO 2022, p. 14)

Of concern, the WHO (2022) suggests that 26% of preventable diseases will be reported in high-income countries between now and 2030 as a direct result of physical inactivity, suggesting that the burden of preventable diseases will be perpetuated rather than reduced. It is also worth noting that women appear to be less active than men (WHO 2022), a point that must be considered when working with childbearing women.

The physiological implications of being inactive for long periods are serious and impact negatively on health from a cellular level in what appear to be otherwise healthy adults. In other words, health is being impacted at a cellular level without the individual's awareness.

The results of inactivity can be summarised as a loss of the body's ability to move properly (hypokinesia) and loss of strength and power in the muscles (hypodynamia); in

DOI: 10.4324/9781003332398-6

addition, adverse modifications to all of the body's systems can be seen (Bergouignan et al. 2011; Le Roux et al. 2022). Being inactive decreases the body's insulin sensitivity, leading to hyperinsulinaemia, and impairs normal glucose disposal. Other, more complex mechanisms are also at play, leading to excess plasma lipids that enhance the development of visceral fat deposits in the muscle, liver and bone (Le Roux et al. 2022). The liver continues to produce glucose, leading to increased hyperinsulinaemia, the end result of which is the development of a continual low-grade inflammation and excessive fat.

Conversely, and as might be expected, being physically active improves the efficiency of every system in the body and reduces the risk of long-term ill health. Bones and muscles are strengthened, suppleness is maintained, the risk of developing an inflammatory status is lower, insulin resistance is reduced (leading to better glycaemic control) and mental health is also improved (Le Roux et al. 2022; WHO 2022). Table 5.1 summarises the benefits for the general population of engaging in physical activity.

It is clear from available evidence that engaging in physical activity is beneficial for all members of society and offers health protection. The WHO (2022) recognises this and presents advice to governments, public health practitioners and health-promoting agents in its Global Action Plan on Physical Activity (GAPPA) report about how to improve the uptake of physical activity for all, including pregnant women, by developing 'enabling environments' where engaging in physical activity becomes 'second nature'. This does not necessarily mean engaging in formal sports events or undertaking coaching or personal training; rather, it entails everyday life tasks. The WHO (2022) defines physical activity as follows:

> Physical activity is defined as any bodily movement produced by skeletal muscle that requires energy expenditure. It can be undertaken in many different ways: walking, cycling, sports and active forms of recreation (such as dance, yoga, tai chi). Physical activity can also be undertaken as part of work (lifting, carrying or other active tasks), and as part of paid or unpaid domestic tasks around the home (cleaning, carrying and care duties).
>
> (WHO 2022, p. 14)

Physical Activity During Pregnancy

For some expectant parents, the thought of engaging in physical activity is not acceptable; there appears to be a belief that to do so will risk harm to the mother or the developing baby or both (Denison et al. 2015; Findley et al. 2020). However, as we have seen,

Table 5.1 Positive impact of engaging in physical activity

'Whole body' benefits	*Benefits to health*
Increased aerobic capacity	Reduced risk of developing cardiovascular disease
Insulin resistance is reduced, leading to Improved glucose control.	Reduced risk of developing type 2 diabetes mellitus (T2DM)
More efficient oxygen uptake for use by muscles	Reduces the risk of developing metabolic syndrome
Reduction in circulating triglycerides levels (the main components of animal fat)	Reduced risk of developing obesity or of its worsening

Source: Adapted from Thyfault and Bergouignan 2020.

engaging in physical activity even at its simplest form can have far-reaching benefits for all individuals in society. This extends to pregnant women, and an emerging body of evidence suggests that engaging in physical activity provides protection rather than posing dangers for both the mother and the developing child.

Benefits of Exercising During Pregnancy

The benefits to obese pregnant women of being physically active mirror the benefits for non-pregnant individuals. Engaging in physical activity during pregnancy has been found to play a part in stabilising maternal weight and limiting gestation weight gain (GWG) (McGiveron et al. 2015; Ronnberg et al. 2015; Haby et al. 2018; Van Poppel 2019; Nagpal & Mottola 2020), which, in turn, has been found to reduce the risk of developing antenatal depression, hypertensive disorders (including pre-eclampsia) and gestational diabetes mellitus (GDM).

Furthermore, engaging in physical activity during pregnancy has been found to be safe for the developing baby, and findings suggest that where a mother does engage in physical activity throughout the pregnancy, the risk of foetal macrosomia is reduced (Kader & Naim-Shuchana 2014), leading to improved outcomes for the baby. There is reduced risk of developing complications such as shoulder dystocia, which can lead to both long- and short-term injury to the baby, foetal hypoglycaemia and early admission to the neonatal unit with its incumbent risks for family bonding.

Professionals therefore have a duty of care to educate *all* pregnant women about the benefits of engaging in physical activity during pregnancy and need to inform them (and family members) that maintaining a level of activity throughout pregnancy and beyond is important for the ongoing health of the woman and her family. However, for those who live with an unhealthy weight, physical activity education is particularly important if the already significant risks to health are to be mitigated.

Professionals who provide care to pregnant women therefore should discuss the benefits of engaging in physical activity at every opportunity during the antenatal course and emphasise the benefits of ongoing physical activity in the postnatal period for the woman and her family members.

Barriers and Facilitators to Physical Activity

The benefits of engaging in physical activity will be achieved only if women become consciously more active, and for those who live with obesity (body mass index [BMI] ≥ 30 kg/m^2), there appear to be complex barriers to doing so, such as issues around body image and a lack of self-confidence (Krans & Chang 2011; Denison et al. 2015). Additional barriers may be at play, such as time constraints, child and other caring responsibilities, the physical challenges of pregnancy (such as bladder issues), lack of awareness about the benefits of exercise, and conflicting advice from friends and family (Denison et al. 2015; Koleilat et al. 2021). Cultural norms that consider engaging in physical activity a danger to the mother or baby may also be a barrier for some women (Krans & Chang 2011) and cause them to have feelings of guilt about potentially harming their baby.

Education Surrounding Physical Activity

When one considers that, for some, lack of awareness about the benefits of engaging in physical activity is a barrier to exercising, this is perhaps a good place to start discussions.

As with other topics discussed in this book, the topic of physical activity needs to be introduced, and a meaningful conversation about it developed between the midwife and the woman. Practitioners need to explore the woman's personal context, allowing her to consider for herself what lifestyle modifications she can make, rather than asking closed questions which often elicit 'yes' or 'no' responses.

During these discussions, women should be provided with evidence about the benefits of engaging in physical activity during pregnancy for her and her unborn baby and the ongoing benefits for the future health of the family. Providing appropriate literature on the topic may also be useful. It is worth noting here that physical activity does not need to be formal or take place in expensive gym venues; it can take any form, from going on a purposeful walk to carrying out activities of daily living (Le Roux et al. 2022; WHO 2022). Indeed, Le Roux et al. (2022) assert that when sedentary behaviours are replaced with movement in daily life, health benefits appear to be more beneficial than when taking part in moderate or vigorous physical activity. This suggests that simple activity that can be fitted in to daily life may be useful for obese pregnant women.

Practical Advice

The WHO (2022) suggests that walking (and cycling) should be promoted as modes of transport. With this in mind and understanding the benefits of engaging in physical activity, it seems appropriate for midwives to advise women to increase their general activity. As with all the topics discussed, the advice needs to take the individual woman's context into account and explore what the woman is able to do to increase her movement.

Examples of how to increase activity time:

- Walking to the local shop rather than driving.
- Parking the car at the furthest parking space from the supermarket door.
- If using public transport, get off the bus at an earlier stop and walk to the destination.
- If out walking, go home 'the long way round'.

If walking is not seen as an option for some, then mobilising in the home should be encouraged. Women should be informed of the risks of sedentary behaviours and advised to maintain mobility by doing household chores and reduce their sedentary times.

Nevertheless, midwives and other healthcare professionals can provide some basic, practical and evidence-based advice about building physical activity into daily life as follows:

Walking – Depending upon fitness level, start with 20-minute walks and build up by 2 minutes per day until walking for 40 minutes. This activity is free and requires no specialist equipment.

Swimming – Depending upon ability, start with 15-minute swim and build up by 2 minutes per session. Cost may exclude some women. Swimming has been found to be less attractive to obese pregnant women because it makes them feel self-conscious (Denison et al. 2015).

Yoga – Attend classes run by a registered yoga teacher or individual educated to provide antenatal yoga classes. Yoga has been found to have several beneficial effects for pregnant women, including reducing the risk of poor mental health, coping well with pain in labour and shortening the length of spontaneous labour (Kwon et al. 2020; Westbury 2019).

It must be borne in mind that if women have been previously inactive, they should *not* be advised to engaged in vigorous physical activity; rather, they should be advised to build episodes gradually in terms of both vigour and length of time over several weeks and months (UK Gov 2019).

Whilst walking is free to do, other activities may be prohibitive for some in terms of cost and this should be borne in mind.

Ongoing Benefits

Engaging in physical activity post-partum is recommended by the UK Government (2019). This will continue to have a beneficial effect on the physical and mental health of the mother, build strength and reduce the risk of intrapartum weight gain. Furthermore, continual engagement in physical activity is likely to set a good example for children and set the family on a good lifelong course.

Contraindications to Physical Activity During Pregnancy

For some, complications do arise in pregnancy that will preclude them from engaging in physical activity or at least curtail their opportunities to do so. It is likely that these individuals will have their pregnancies monitored and managed by obstetricians and other appropriate specialists who oversee 'high risk' antenatal clinics and that midwives will not be their primary healthcare provider. Nevertheless, midwives and other professionals need to be in possession of accurate knowledge if they are to appropriately advise women about the benefits of engaging in physical activity. Table 5.2 provides an overview of the conditions that may preclude women from engaging in physical activity during pregnancy.

Table 5.2 Absolute contraindications to vigorous exercise

Conditions that preclude physical activity	*Professional support*
Severe cardiac and/or respiratory disease Cervical incompetence/cerclage Placenta praevia After 26 weeks' gestation where there is placenta praevia Persistent vaginal bleeding Premature labour in current pregnancy Pre-term rupture of the membranes	Women who have these conditions should be carefully monitored and advised by appropriate clinicians.
Some relative conditions that urge caution around physical activity	
Severe iron deficiency anaemia Severe chronic respiratory disease Pregnancy-related hypertensive disorders Growth restricted baby in the current pregnancy Poorly controlled diabetes, thyroid disease or seizure disorder	These conditions need to be carefully reviewed and managed and appropriate advice given to women who develop these conditions but also live with an unhealthy weight.
Warning signs to women about when to stop exercising	
Vaginal bleeding Breathlessness prior to exercising Dizziness, headaches or chest pains Calf pain (may be a deep vein thrombosis) Reduced foetal movement	The attending professional needs to exercise critical thinking and advise women about where to seek ongoing professional review.

Sources: Adapted from Kader & Naim-Shuchana 2014; Brook 2017.

The table above summarises some conditions that may preclude some women from engaging in physical activity; however, depending upon the woman's individual context, some gentle exercise may be acceptable. Midwives therefore need to demonstrate that they are knowledgeable and are in possession of the appropriate information about physical activity when working with overweight and obese pregnant women. The advice these women should receive will depend on their individual context and the severity of the condition or complication they are experiencing as well as the gestation at which these occur. Advice should be sought from specialist clinicians about their ongoing medical management and about what may be acceptable exercise levels during a complex pregnancy.

Conclusion

This chapter has provided an overview of the importance and benefits of engaging in physical activity during pregnancy. Women who live with an unhealthy weight can improve their health and potentially optimise pregnancy outcomes. However, advice needs to be developed and imparted with the individual context being borne in mind and should be achievable for each individual. Now consider the questions posed in Box 5.1 and consider how your knowledge about pregnancy and physical activity may influence your practice.

Box 5.1 Professional Reflective Questions

- Consider the knowledge you previously had about engaging in physical activity during pregnancy.
  - Reflect on the knowledge that you have with respect to physical activity. Has your perspective on the topic changed?
  - From what sources did you acquire this knowledge and information about physical activity during pregnancy?
  - Was it from professional sources or the general media, for example?
  - What resources and sources have been most useful for you?
  - Consider how much emphasis you placed on the topic of physical activity when working with women. How will your practice now change?
- Now consider how you raised the topic of physical activity, particularly with women who live with an unhealthy weight.
  - Were the institutional questionnaires influential? Did they enable or disable the initiation of conversations around engaging in physical activity?
  - Consider how you explore women's physical activity levels with them. Will you now change this as your practice develops?
- Now that you have read this chapter and Chapter 1, consider how you might start to develop a meaningful conversation about engaging in physical activity.
  - Consider how you will discern an individual's personal context with respect to their intention to engage in physical activity.
  - Consider what questions or statements you might use when initiating and continuing a conversation about physical activity.

References

Bergouignan, A., Rudwill, F, Simon, C., & Blanc, S. (2011). Physical inactivity as the culprit of metabolic inflexibility: Evidence of bedrest studies. *Journal of Applied Physiology*, *111*(4), 1201–1210. https://doi.org/10.1152/japplphysiol.00698.2011

Brook, G. (2017). Physical preparation for childbirth and beyond, and the role of the physiotherapy. In S. Macdonald and G. Johnson (Eds). *Mayes' Midwifery* (15th ed, pp. 331–343). Elsevier.

Denison, W. Z., Carver, H., Norman, J. E., & Reynolds, R. M. (2015). Physical activity in pregnant women with Class III obesity: A qualitative exploration of attitudes and behaviours. *Midwifery*, *31*(12), 1163–1167. https://doi.org/10.1016/j.midw.2015.08.006

Findley, A., Smith, D. M., Hesketh, K., & Keyworth, C. (2020). Exploring women's experiences and decision making about physical activity during pregnancy and following birth: A qualitative study. *BMC Pregnancy and Childbirth*, *20*(1), 54–54. https://doi.org/10.1186/s12884-019-2707-7

Haby, K., Berg, M., Gyllensten, H., Hanas, R., & Premberg, Å. (2018). Mighty Mums – A lifestyle intervention at primary care level reduces gestational weight gain in women with obesity. *BMC Obesity*, *5*(1), 16. https://doi.org/10.1186/s40608-018-0194-4

Kader, M., & Naim-Shuchana, S. (2014). Physical activity during pregnancy. *European Journal of Physiotherapy*, *16*(1), 2–9. http://doi.org/10.3109/21679169.2013.861509

Koleilat, V. N., vanTwist, V., & Kodjebacheva, G. D. (2021). Perceived barriers to and suggested interventions for physical activity during pregnancy among participants of the Special Supplemental Nutrition Program for Women, Infants, and Children (WIC) in Southern California. *BMC Pregnancy and Childbirth*, *21*(1), 69–69. https://doi.org/10.1186/s12884-021-03553-7

Krans, E. E., & Chang, J. C. (2011). A will without a way: Barriers and facilitators to exercise during pregnancy of low-income, African American women. *Women & Health*, *51*(8), 777–794. https://doi.org/10.1080/03630242.2011.633598

Kwon, R., Kasper, K., London, S., & Hass, D. M. (2020). A systematic review: The effects of yoga on pregnancy. *European Journal of Obstetrics, Gynaecology and Reproductive Biology*, *250*, 171–177. https://doi.org/10.1016/j.ejogrb.2020.03.044

Le Roux, E., De Jong, N. P., Blanc, S., Simon, C., Bessesen, D. H., & Bergouignan, A. (2022). Physiology of physical inactivity, sedentary behaviours and non-exercise activity: Insights from the space bedrest model. *The Journal of Physiology*, *600*(5), 1037–1051. https://doi.org/10.1113/JP281064

McGiveron, F. S., Pearce, J., Taylor, M. A., McMullen, S., & Langley-Evans, S. C. (2015). Limiting antenatal weight gain improves maternal health outcomes in severely obese pregnant women: Findings of a pragmatic evaluation of a midwife-led intervention. *Journal of Human Nutrition and Dietetics*, *28*(s1), 29–37. https://doi.org/10.1111/jhn.12240

Nagpal, T. S., & Mottola, M. F. (2020). Physical activity throughout pregnancy is key to preventing chronic disease. *Reproduction (Cambridge, England)*, *160*(5), R111–R118. https://doi.org/10.1530/REP-20-0337

Ronnberg, A. K., Ostlund, I., Fadl, H., Gottvall, T., & Nilsson, K. (2015). Intervention during pregnancy to reduce excessive gestational weight gain—A randomised controlled trial. *BJOG: An International Journal of Obstetrics and Gynaecology*, *122*(4), 537–544. https://doi.org/10.1111/1471-0528.13131

Thyfault, & Bergouignan, A. (2020). Exercise and metabolic health: Beyond skeletal muscle. *Diabetologia*, *63*(8), 1464–1474. https://doi.org/10.1007/s00125-020-05177-6

UK Government. (2019). Physical activity guidelines: Pregnancy and after childbirth. Retrieved from https://www.gov.uk/government/publications/physical-activity-guidelines-pregnancy-and-after-childbirth

van Poppel, M., Owe, K. M., Santos-Rocha, R., & Dias, H. (2019). Physical activity, exercise and health promotion for the pregnant exerciser and pregnant athlete. In R. Santos-Rocha (Ed.), *Exercise and sporting activity during pregnancy* (1st ed., pp. 1–17). Springer. https://doi.org/10.1007/978-3-319-91032-1_1

Westbury. B. (2019). Measuring the benefits of free pregnancy yoga classes. *British Journal of Midwifery*, 27(2), 100–105. https://doi.org/10.12968/bjom.2019.27.2.100

World Health Organization. (2022). Global status report on physical activity 2022. https://www.who.int/teams/health-promotion/physical-activity/global-status-report-on-physical-activity-2022

6 The Evidence Around Diet and Physical Activity During Pregnancy

Introduction

Throughout this book, there has been discussion about the value of providing obese women with both dietary and physical activity advice that, if followed, is likely to support them in maintaining and stabilising their weight throughout pregnancy. This has been found to optimise health and improve pregnancy outcomes.

This chapter provides a short review of some of the evidence that pertains to lifestyle interventions that can improve health and pregnancy outcomes for obese women.

The Evidence

Interest in 'obese pregnancy' became dominant in the literature from about 2010, although some papers were published prior to this. Anecdotally, it was becoming obvious that more women were presenting for maternity care with a raised body mass index (BMI) of more than 30 kg/m^2 and this inevitably generated discussion and debate amongst clinicians about the effect of obesity on the woman and the baby and the impact upon staff of caring for women with raised BMI, and the overall additional costs of providing women with safe care were also commonly discussed in maternity care settings.

Many studies have been published about the impact of living with obesity from a scientific and medical perspective and have observed physiological changes from a cellular level to a psychosocial one. In addition, interest has grown with respect to how lifestyle changes in obese women might affect both the mother's and the unborn baby's health.

An Overview of Some Key Studies

Between 2014 and 2019, several key papers were published with respect to lifestyle interventions during pregnancy where the mother was obese. A summary of them can be seen in Table 6.1.

In all of the studies mentioned, dietary and lifestyle advice was provided for women. This was done in a variety of ways, in either group or individual sessions, prescribing physical activity or informing women verbally about how they could improve their lifestyles by increasing fruit and vegetable intake and engaging in physical activity. The information was provided by trained or specialist midwives, research assistants or nutritional specialists. In all cases where women engaged with the advice given, there appeared to be a reduction in GWG, no adverse outcomes for the babies were seen, and there

DOI: 10.4324/9781003332398-7

Table 6.1 Summary of studies exploring lifestyle changes during obese pregnancy

Authors, date and country	*Title*	*Interventions*	*Outcomes*
Dodd et al. (2016) Australia	The effect of antenatal dietary and lifestyle advice for women who are overweight or obese on emotional wellbeing: The LIMIT randomized trial	Dietary and exercise advice given to women by a research dietitian and a trained research assistant versus standard care	Knowledge about health food choices and physical activity improved but did not negatively impact on wellbeing.
Dodd et al. (2014) Australia	Antenatal lifestyle advice for women who are overweight or obese: LIMIT randomised trial	Dietary and exercise advice given to women by a research dietitian and a trained research assistant versus standard care	The risk of large for dates infants being born is not reduced, nor are maternal health outcomes affected.
Jewell (2014) UK	The healthy eating and lifestyle in pregnancy (HELP) feasibility study	Available to women with body mass index (BMI) of 30 kg/m^2 or more. Dietary advice provided by specialist midwife and Slimming World consultant.	An acceptable intervention for women. Babies born to women who lost weight were more likely to be born within a normal weight range.
McGiveron et al. (2015) UK	Limiting antenatal weight gain improves maternal health outcomes in severely obese pregnant women: findings of a pragmatic evaluation of a midwife-led intervention	All women with a BMI > 35 kg/m^2 were offered a meeting with a lifestyle advisor or midwife. Eight sessions were offered throughout pregnancy and postnatally.	Overall, there was a lower rate of pregnancy complications when women engaged in the advice given. A significant reduction in hypertension complications was seen.
Ronnberg et al. (2015) Sweden	Intervention during pregnancy to reduce excessive gestational weight gain—a randomised controlled trial	Standard care versus personalised prescription of exercise, regular weighing and monitoring of gestational weight gain (GWG)	The mean GWG was lower, but a proportion of women exceeded weight gain above the Institute of Medicine (IOM) guidance.
Haby et al. (2018) Sweden	Mighty Mums—an antenatal healthcare intervention can reduce gestational weight gain in women with obesity	A randomised controlled trial. Standard care versus an intervention consisting of individualised dietary advice and prescribed physical activity. Food discussion groups were also offered.	Women who engaged with the intervention had lower GWG and have less risk of retaining weight after birth.
Hayes (2015) UK	Change in level of physical activity during pregnancy in obese women: findings from the UK Pregnancies Better Eating and Activity Trial (UPBEAT) pilot trial	A study aimed at comparing physical activity and glycaemic control throughout pregnancy where women lived with BMI 30 kg/m^2. Objective assessment of physical activity was monitored throughout pregnancy.	Physical activity should be encouraged in women prior to conception, and they should be advised to continue this throughout pregnancy. Advice should be tailored to suit the needs of the woman.

appeared to be improved health for the mothers with less incidence of hypertensive complications and gestational diabetes mellitus (GDM). However, as Langley-Evans (2022) points out, the success of these studies is somewhat dependent upon the women who take part in engaging with advice and it is likely that those who did participate were motivated to follow any advice given.

Langley-Evans et al. (2022) also urge caution when interpreting the results of these randomised controlled trials (RCTs) pertaining to nutrition and suggest that some women may fail to see any benefit of choosing nutritionally valuable foods and revert to normal (unhealthy) food choices. Women in control groups may have chosen of more nutritional value too when they learn about the study, causing bias in results.

Another word of caution, however, is that of the population being studied. For example, in the 'Bumps and Beyond' intervention study by McGiveron et al. (2015), less than 50% of the woman invited to take part accepted. This suggests that, for some, any advice given pertaining to weight management or lifestyle may not be acceptable, practical or affordable and that such families who decline that advice may be living in situations of deprivation. These socioeconomic and psychosocial issues need to be considered when reviewing such papers since individuals who may benefit from practical nutritional advice and physical activity advice may be 'hard to reach' and therefore 'omitted' from any research populations.

Systematic Reviews

Since the publication of the above studies, several systematic reviews have been published (Magro-Malossa et al. [2017], Dalrymple et al. [2018], Flannery et al. [2019]). The number of papers included in each review was low: nine, eighteen and nineteen (three of which were described narratively) respectively. Magro-Malossa et al. (2017) and Flannery et al. (2019) both reviewed the effect of exercise during pregnancy, and Magro-Malossa et al. (2017) specifically reviewed studies pertaining to the risk of preterm birth. Dalrymple et al. (2018) reviewed papers with respect to weight management either during or following pregnancy.

Magro-Molossa et al. (2017) found that women who exercised were less at risk of preterm birth. They concluded that women who live with an unhealthy weight should be counselled about engaging in physical activity for 30 to 60 minutes three to seven times per week. Complementing these findings, Flannery et al. (2019) concluded that specific strategies should be utilised in order for women to monitor their own progress, such as 'goal setting', 'feedback and monitoring', 'knowledge shaping' and identifying 'social support'. Findings from Dalrymple et al. (2018) suggest that interventions for postpartum weight management may be effective; however, they go on to say that more evidence is required to understand how long-term weight maintenance can be achieved. It would appear, according to the evidence reviewed, that when women engage in physical activity and are monitored and given 'goals' and feedback their pregnancy outcomes are improved and that engaging in lifestyle changes following birth is effective in controlling post-partum weight gain.

The Cochrane Review undertaken by Shepherd et al. (2017) to explore whether lifestyle interventions impacted on a GDM diagnosis found that there was considerable diversity in the studies reviewed (n = 39). They concluded that risks of GDM and Caesarean section were reduced when there was a combination of diet and exercise interventions resulting in reduced GWG. However, they also note that there was little difference in other outcomes such as hypertensive complications, perinatal mortality, perineal trauma, the birth of macrosomic babies, and neonatal hypoglycaemia. They note that the quality of studies was 'moderate to very low'. They go on to say that any future studies need to describe in more detail the interventions reported upon and how behaviour change in women was influenced. Nevertheless, the current evidence does suggest that when women improve diet and increase physical activity, the risks of poor pregnancy outcomes are reduced.

Additional Literature

There is now a plethora of literature available in the major academic databases that report upon obese pregnancy, the impact of obesity on mothers and babies during pregnancy, and the benefits of lifestyle interventions with respect to diet and physical activity. In addition, evidence continues to emerge with respect to the impact of obese pregnancy on the offspring born to obese women throughout the lifelong continuum. Despite these many publications, an effective lifestyle intervention aimed at improving diet and physical activity for obese women to improve pregnancy outcomes and overall maternal and child health has not been universally agreed. Many studies appear to be observational and of low quality (Shepherd et al. [2017]). However, Mills et al. (2019), as part of the UPBEAT study, did measure biochemical markers throughout pregnancy where lifestyle intervention was advised and found that there were beneficial effects in women's glycaemic control and fatty acid profiles. These objective biochemical markers are unequivocal and demonstrate that positive changes to lifestyle are effective in improving the health of mothers and babies. What is less clear, however, is how to reach all women who live with an unhealthy weight, counsel them effectively and persuade them to engage in making positive lifestyle changes.

The few studies presented here vary in quality and robustness with respect to research design, populations being studied, and the interventions themselves. More work is therefore required to explore what the optimal professional approach might be when providing advice with the aim of motivating women who live with raised BMI > 30 kg/m^2 to change their dietary and physical activity habits. Professional practice with respect to giving advice in a positive manner will also be useful.

Conclusion

This chapter has provided an overview of some of the key studies that have been reported upon with respect to lifestyle interventions for women who live with an unhealthy weight. The studies presented are not exhaustive, and it would be advisable to read further about this topic. Nevertheless, one can discern from these papers that engaging women who live with unhealthy weights in conversations about their lifestyles and diet and encouraging changes can be of value in order to promote good health and optimal pregnancy outcomes. This brings us full circle and suggests that to be able to provide lifestyle advice effectively, good consultation skills are required to initiate and maintain honest and effective conversations between women and healthcare professionals. Now consider the following questions in Box 6.1. How might your knowledge about lifestyle choices influence your practice?

Box 6.1 Professional Reflective Questions

- In the course of your practice, consider how knowledgeable you have been with respect to the evidence that surrounds the impact of lifestyle behaviour change.
  - What motivates you to read the evidence with respect to this topic?
  - How do you currently answer women's questions prior to having additional knowledge about this subject area?
  - How might you now move forward in your practice with respect to additional reading? (What might your specific responses be if a woman asked you what the risks of obesity during pregnancy are?)
- Consider how important it is to engage with the evidence prior to meeting a woman with specific needs.
  - How important do you consider reading original evidence to be in addition to reading, knowing and understanding the local policies and protocols?
  - How might you overcome any barriers that you perceive when you attempt to read any original evidence?
- Consider how often you critically reflect upon your practice in response to the evidence base.
  - How do you strive to model your practice on the evidence that you have read rather than relying upon local protocols and policies?
- Consider a recent consultation episode that you have facilitated and formally reflect upon it.
  - Consider how you might use any published evidence with respect to lifestyle changes when holding conversations with women about their food and physical activity choices.

References

Dalrymple, K. V., Flynn, A. C., Relph, S. A., O'Keeffe, M., & Poston, L. (2018). Lifestyle interventions in overweight and obese pregnant or postpartum women for postpartum weight management: A systematic review of the literature. *Nutrients*, *10*(11), 1704. https://doi.org/10.3390/nu10111704

Dodd, J., Newman, A., Moran, L. J., Deussen, A. R., Grivell, R. M., Yelland, L. N., Crowther, C. A., McPhee, A. J., Wittert, G., Owens, J. A., Turnbull, D., & Robinson, J. S. (2016). The effect of antenatal dietary and lifestyle advice for women who are overweight or obese on emotional well-being: The LIMIT randomized trial. *Acta Obstetricia et Gynecologica Scandinavica*, *95*(3), 309–318. https://doi.org/10.1111/aogs.12832

Dodd, J., Turnbull, D., McPhee, A. J., Deussen, A. R., Grivell, R. M., Yelland, L. N., Crowther, C. A., Wittert, G., Owens, J. A., & Robinson, J. S. (2014). Antenatal lifestyle advice for women who are overweight or obese: LIMIT randomised trial. *British Medical Journal (Online)*, *348*, 285–1285. https://doi.org/10.1136/bmj.g1285

Flannery, C., Fredrix, M., Olander, E. K., McAuliffe, F. M., Byrne, M., & Kearney, P. M. (2019). Effectiveness of physical activity interventions for overweight and obesity during pregnancy: A systematic review of the content of behaviour change interventions. *The International Journal of Behavioral Nutrition and Physical Activity*, *16*(1), 97–97. https://doi.org/10.1186/s12966-019-0859-5

Haby, K., Berg, M., Gyllensten, H., Hanas, R., & Premberg, Å. (2018). Mighty Mums – A lifestyle intervention at primary care level reduces gestational weight gain in women with obesity. *BMC Obesity*, *5*(1), 16. https://doi.org/10.1186/s40608-018-0194-4

Hayes, L., Mcparlin, C., Kinnunen, T. I., Poston, L., Robson, S. C., & Bell, R. (2015). Change in level of physical activity during pregnancy in obese women: Findings from the UPBEAT pilot trial. *BMC Pregnancy and Childbirth*, *15*(1), 52. https://doi.org/10.1186/s12884-015-0479-2

Jewell, K., Avery, A., Barber, J., & Simpson, S. (2014). The healthy eating and lifestyle in pregnancy (HELP) feasibility study. *British Journal of Midwifery*, *22*(10), 727–736. https://doi.org/10.12968/bjom.2014.22.10.727

Langley-Evans, S. C., Pearce, J., & Ellis, S. (April, 2022). Overweight, obesity and excessive weight gain in pregnancy as risk factors for adverse pregnancy outcomes: A narrative review. *Journal of Human Nutrition and Dietetics*, *35*(2), 250–264. https://doi.org/10.1111/jhn.12999

Magro-Malosso, E. R., Saccone, G., Di Mascio, D., Di Tommaso, M., & Berghella, V. (2017). Exercise during pregnancy and risk of preterm birth in overweight and obese women: A systematic review and meta-analysis of randomized controlled trials. *Acta Obstetricia et Gynecologica Scandinavica*, *96*(3), 263–273. https://doi.org/10.1111/aogs.13087

McGiveron, A., Foster, S., Pearce, J., Taylor, M. A., McMullen, S., & Langley-Evans, S. C. (2015). Limiting antenatal weight gain improves maternal health outcomes in severely obese pregnant women: Findings of a pragmatic evaluation of a midwife-led intervention. *Journal of Human Nutrition and Dietetics*, *28*(s1), 29–37. https://doi.org/10.1111/jhn.12240

Mills, H. L., Patel, N., White, S. L., Pasupathy, D., Briley, A. L., Ferreira, D. L. S., Seed, P. T., Nelson, S. M., Sattar, N., Tilling, K., Poston, L., & Lawlor, D. A. (2019). The effect of a lifestyle intervention in obese pregnant women on gestational metabolic profiles: Findings from the UK Pregnancies Better Eating and Activity Trial (UPBEAT) randomised controlled trial. *BMC Medicine*, *17*(1), 15–15. https://doi.org/10.1186/s12916-018-1248-7

Ronnberg, A. K., Ostlund, I., Fadl, H., Gottvall, T., & Nilsson, K. (2015). Intervention during pregnancy to reduce excessive gestational weight gain—A randomised controlled trial. *BJOG: An International Journal of Obstetrics and Gynaecology*, *122*(4), 537–544. https://doi.org/10.1111/1471-0528.13131

Shepherd, E., Gomersall, J. C., Tieu, J., Han, S., Crowther, C. A., & Middleton, P. (2017). Combined diet and exercise interventions for preventing gestational diabetes mellitus. *Cochrane Database of Systematic Reviews*, *11*(11), CD010443. https://doi.org/10.1002/14651858.CD010443.pub3

7 Additional Considerations

Introduction

This final chapter discusses additional issues that are pertinent to maternity care and public health. It discusses the benefits of, and the case for, providing pre-conceptual care and also some of the challenges around its provision, particularly for women who live with an unhealthy weight. The topic of eating disorders is also briefly discussed with the understanding that midwives need to have an awareness of these illnesses and the appropriate referral pathways that will ensure safe care. A comprehensive discussion about eating disorders and their treatment is beyond the scope of this book; however, some brief information has been included.

The Concept of Pre-Conceptual Care?

Pre-conceptual care is concerned with optimising health prior to conception. Prospective parents should be provided with evidence-based information pertaining to their current lifestyle choices so that they have the opportunity to change behaviours where appropriate and, where they live with obesity, to optimise their body mass index (BMI). Theoretically, this has a two-pronged effect: to reduce the risk of experiencing complications during pregnancy, labour and birth and in the postnatal period and to set the child and family on a healthy lifelong course (Brooke-Read & Burden 2017). The three principal areas that span this concept are risk assessment, lifestyle education, and behaviour change and/or lifestyle interventions (Brooke-Read & Burden 2017). De Leo et al. (2022) suggest that the 'pre-conceptual' period is a window of opportunity to promote health that is underutilised. However, there appears to be a general lack of awareness of the availability of these services in the UK (De Leo et al. 2022), suggesting that even if people would find this health promotion approach valuable, they wouldn't actively seek services. A vicious circle has therefore developed. It is of concern that some women who live with unhealthy lifestyle habits such as smoking or, as is the focus here, obesity may conceive and raise their families having not had the opportunity to receive evidence-based information about the risks of obesity (and other lifestyle choices), suggesting that the cycle of obesity is likely to continue.

Pre-Conceptual Care – The Challenges

Currently in the UK context, pre-conceptual care is not part of the 'routine' suite of services offered by the National Health Service (NHS) with the exception of those who already live with pre-existing medical conditions such as hypertension, diabetes or

DOI: 10.4324/9781003332398-8

epilepsy. Other groups who may receive appropriate pre-conceptual counselling are parents who may have had a poor pregnancy outcome such as stillbirth, neonatal death or a very sick baby who has been required to remain in the neonatal unit for many days, weeks or months (Brooke-Read & Burden 2017) and women who have suffered from morbidity following pregnancy and birth. However, the content of these consultations usually occurs with senior medical staff, and the focus of these consultations is likely to be upon how future pregnancies and births will be monitored and managed. It is not clear how much information about health promotion and lifestyle changes is discussed at such appointments.

Whilst it is optimal for these families to receive this medical attention, there is likely to remain a large population of women who will not seek any type of pre-conceptual advice, believing that they are fit and well despite their current lifestyle choices. One must also bear in mind that the decision to plan a pregnancy is likely to be a private one and this may have a bearing on whether pre-conceptual advice is sought by women or families irrespective of their health and lifestyle choices.

Challenges with Providing the Service

Public Health England (PHE) (2018) makes a strong case for providing pre-conceptual care and recognises that supporting women to adopt health behaviours can reduce risk of poor pregnancy outcomes occurring to mothers and babies. However, the debate about who should provide this care and where it should be provided continues, particularly in a climate where all healthcare professional groups have competing demands (PHE 2019).

Whilst general practitioners (GPs), midwives and Health Visitors (HVs) appear to be the best placed professional groups to deliver this advice because of their community-based situation, there are competing priorities in all three professions suggesting that to ‘add on’ a pre-conceptual clinic may be an unachievable commitment. However, it is now recognised that pre-conceptual care should be provided in a more holistic manner and the design of such services should include professional groups, third sector charities and social policy makers and have an ‘all inclusive’ approach in society (Tuomainen et al. 2013). However, funding debates and challenges will no doubt continue. Nevertheless, it would be worthwhile to consider the benefits of providing comprehensive pre-conceptual care and the benefits of supporting people to optimise their health and the eventual healthcare cost savings that are, in the longer term, likely to be made.

The discussion above has focused on women who may be planning their first pregnancy. However, GPs, midwives and HVs can provide good-quality pre-conceptual advice in the postnatal period (midwives and HVs) and in the longer term when they meet with families over time (GPs and HVs).

Pre-Conceptual Care and Obesity

With respect to obesity, women, prior to conception, should generally receive the same advice that their pregnant counterparts receive: to improve diet quality and to increase physical activity. However, they should also be advised to optimise their BMI prior to conception because, as discussed earlier, these women have poorer chances of conceiving and are likely to have impaired glucose tolerance and be at risk of miscarriage, pre-eclampsia, venous thromboembolism (VTE) disease and, worryingly, a high risk of maternal death (PHE 2019). Women should be given realistic goals about their targets, and plans should be made in discussion with them. It may be advantageous for women to be followed-up and appointments made that are of most use to them, in keeping with the continuity-of-care philosophy of midwifery practice (Scottish Government 2017: NHS England 2017).

It is likely that investing in pre-conceptual services will be a positive step with respect to health promotion; however, it cannot be taken for granted that individuals will access services. De Leo et al. (2022), in their review, found that the main influencers and sources of information for young women considering pregnancy were their friends and family. Given these findings, it may be some years before pre-conceptual care is fully integrated into UK systems and we begin to see any significant difference in women's preparation for pregnancy and in turn a reduction in BMI levels amongst young childbearing women.

Eating Disorders

The term 'eating disorders' is an umbrella term used to describe mental health illnesses that result in individuals having an 'unhealthy' relationship with food and having altered eating behaviours (Bye et al. 2018). A summary of these can be seen in Table 7.1.

Eating disorders can affect women at any time in life, but most commonly they develop between the ages of 13 and 17 years (NICE 2017), meaning that some childbearing women may present for care who have already lived with an eating disorder for some

Table 7.1 Summary of eating disorders

Eating Disorder	*Symptoms*
Anorexia nervosa (AN)	• The individual persistently restricts food which ultimate leads to a low weight and eventually the body is starved. • The individual develops an intense fear of gaining weight. • The individual develops a distorted view of their body weight and shape.
Bulimia nervosa (BM)	• The individual experiences episodes of binge eating where they eat excessive amounts of food and are unable to control what and when they eat. • A binge episode is followed by compensatory behaviour where the individual fasts, may misuse laxatives or engages in excessive physical activity. • Body weight and shape have a disproportionate influence on self-worth. • This occurs at least once per week for a three-month period. • People who suffer from this type of disorder do not necessarily have a low body mass index (BMI).
Binge eating disorders	• This has similarities to BM, but the individual does not follow a binge episode with compensatory behaviour. • The individual may eat rapidly, eat large volumes of food in the absence of hunger or eat alone to 'hide' their eating problem. • Binge eating will cause the individual emotional distress following the event. • Similar to BM, this occurs at least once per week for a period of 3 months or more.
Other specified feeding or eating disorder (OSFED)	• This category includes other non-specific conditions where they become distressed as a result of their eating behaviours, but their symptoms do not meet the criteria for AN, BM or binge eating.

Sources: Adapted from Bye et al. 2018.

time; for others, it may be a relatively new healthcare problem. Midwives do not need to be experts in the field of eating disorders, but they do need an awareness of what they are and how suffering from one can cause significant risk to women and their babies. Therefore, they need to be vigilant when exploring the topics of diet and nutrition with all women and ensure that, in the context of the antenatal consultation, they ask appropriate open-ended questions in order to screen for such conditions. All women need to be screened for such illnesses, but particular focus regarding these conditions should be put on those with a significantly high or low BMI (<18.5 kg/m^2 or >35 kg/m^2).

Risks of Eating Disorders During Pregnancy

Significant risks exist for women and babies where a woman has an eating disorder. Where a woman has AN, there is significant risk of foetal growth restriction and a high incidence of Caesarean section birth (Pan et al. 2022). However, Linna et al. (2014) found that those who suffered from binge eating disorders were more at risk of living with a raised BMI and being exposed to similar risks to those who lived with obesity but didn't have an eating disorder. In an older study, Bulik et al. (2009) found that women with binge eating disorders were more likely to need induction of labour, give birth to large for gestational age (LGA) babies and require Caesarean section.

The findings of these studies suggest that women who live with a raised BMI may have also been living with an eating disorder of some type. For these reasons, the topic should not be shied away from by professionals, and midwives should not shy away from including the topic during antenatal consultation periods. Consultation episodes should facilitate a careful and detailed discussion not only about the woman's nutritional intake but also about her eating behaviours.

It should be noted that, for some, talking about this topic can be difficult and distressing and that the woman may feel that she is being shamed or stigmatised (NICE 2017). Nevertheless, if an eating disorder is suspected or indeed disclosed to the midwife, then he/she must act upon and ensure that appropriate care is put in place for the woman and her family. The midwife also needs to discuss in detail with the woman what the risks are to her and her baby, not to cause fear but to demonstrate that the aim of the pregnancy is to keep both mother and child safe.

The principles of care for those who suffer from eating disorders are to provide continuous support by a dedicated professional (NICE 2017) who can support the woman throughout pregnancy and birth and in the postnatal period. In the context of maternity care, this aligns with the 'continuity of carer' philosophy (NMC 2019) where the woman has her care provided by one midwife or a small group of midwives. However, collaboration with specialists will also be required if robust and consistent care is to be provided.

Referrals to Specialists

Women and babies are at risk when the expectant mother suffers from an eating disorder. As with other high-risk pregnancies, care should be taken to make appropriate referrals to specialists so that robust care can be provided. The woman should be informed in detail about the potential risks she faces and the rationale for making referrals to obstetricians, psychiatrists, dietitians or other specialists who can offer support throughout the pregnancy. However, the woman needs to be at the centre of her own care and involved in any decision making. Her consent should be sought and given before any ongoing referrals are made (NMC 2019). Midwives also need to have an awareness of the care provision available for such women within their health authority or geographical area.

Postnatal Care

The risks for women who live with eating disorders continue following birth and this poses an additional layer of risk for those who already live with a BMI level at either end of the spectrum. The risks of VTE disease, infection, poor breastfeeding rates, and anxiety and depression have all been found to increase where a woman has lived with an eating disorder (Bye et al. 2018; Martinez-Olcina et al. 2020).

It is important that the relationship that is built up between the woman and the midwife antenatally continue into the postnatal phase. There is an increased risk that symptoms of the eating disorder will resume postnatally (Stringer & Furber 2019), and it is anticipated that a positive midwife–woman relationship will put the expectant mother at ease and make it easier for her to disclose if this is the case or not. The midwife should act upon any concerns he/she may have about the woman and ensure that appropriate care is provided.

Care of the woman will be transferred to other professionals a few weeks following the birth and so it is incumbent upon the midwife to engage in collaborative practice and adequately inform colleagues from other disciplines about the woman's situation: her history, the relationship she has with the baby and other family members, how she is feeling and how she is coping with her pre-existing eating disorder. Key professionals in the UK who will be involved in providing ongoing care are HVs and GPs. In some cases, psychiatric and dietetic care may already be in place. However, Pan et al. (2022) recommend that all women who have suffered from AN during pregnancy should be followed up during the postnatal period because of the high risk of symptoms worsening following birth.

Conclusion

This concluding chapter has discussed some of the wider concerns with respect to maternity care.

Pre-conceptual care may be of benefit for some women and support them to prepare for pregnancy and optimise their health. This is likely to require significant investment by health authorities, and challenges exist with respect to accommodation, the professionals who should provide it and whether women will access such a service. There is now recognition that this topic can be provided in a holistic manner and that pre-conceptual care should be provided by wider community organisations and by all healthcare professionals.

Eating disorders have also been discussed. These are serious mental health issues, and altered eating and sub-optimal nutritional intake can adversely affect the pregnancy. Midwives need to have an awareness of these conditions and develop the skills to appropriately screen for them during antenatal consultations. They also need to have a working knowledge of the care provision that is available for women in their health authority area and how to make appropriate referrals to it. Now please consider the professional reflective questions in Box 7.1.

Box 7.1 Professional Reflective Questions

- In the course of your practice, have you met any woman who has accessed pre-conceptual care?
  - How did accessing such care appear to influence her knowledge?
  - In your opinion, what difference did this make (if any) to the communication between the midwife and the woman?
  - In your opinion, was the woman influenced to make lifestyle changes that may have optimised her health during pregnancy as a result of pre-conceptual advice?
- During the course of your professional practice, have you met with women who you believe may have benefitted from accessing pre-conceptual care?
  - Taking the woman's personal context into account, how do you think this service could have been provided for women with respect to their social and financial context?
  - What other professionals may have been able to provide the necessary care to support the woman to optimise her health prior to pregnancy?
- Consider whether you have come across any women who may have been suffering from an eating disorder during your practice.
  - What questions did you ask with respect to this whilst providing care?
  - Now on reflection, how effective do think these questions were in assessing the woman's eating behaviours?
  - How might you explore this topic with women as your practice develops?
- If you have provided care for a woman who has been suffering from an eating disorder, consider the following questions.
  - Were you aware prior to the midwifery consultation that the woman suffered from this illness? If so, how was the information conveyed?
  - Consider what communication pathways may have been beneficial for you in learning of the woman's illness.
  - Consider what you could suggest to your health authority that may improve information sharing with respect to maternity care and eating disorders.

Reflect upon how you managed the situation and what other professionals you referred the woman to. What might you do differently if faced with a similar situation in the future?

References

Brooke-Read, M., & Burden, B. (2017). Preconception care. In S. Macdonald & G. Johnson (Eds.), *Mayes' midwifery* (15th ed., pp. 303–317). Elsevier.

Bulik, C. M., Von Holle, A., Siega-Riz, A. M., Torgersen, L., Lie, K. K., Hamer, R. M., Berg, C. K., Sullivan, P., & Reichborn-Kjennerud, T. (2009). Birth outcomes in women with eating disorders in the Norwegian mother and child cohort study (MoBa). *The International Journal of Eating Disorders*, *42*(1), 9–18. https://doi.org/10.1002/eat.20578

Bye, A., Mackintosh, N., Sandall, J., Easter, A., & Walker, M. (2018). Supporting women with eating disorders during pregnancy and the postnatal period. *Journal of Health Visiting*, *6*(5), 224–228. https://doi.org/10.12968/johv.2018.6.5.224

De Leo, A., Neesham, B. M. Bepete, N., Mukaro, A., Nepal, B. T., N'geno, C., & Muhandiramalag, T. A. (2022). Engaging in pre-conceptual care: An integrative review. *British Journal of Midwifery*, *30*(11), 644–651. https://doi.org/10.12968/bjom.2022.30.11.644

Eating Disorders: Recognition and Treatment [NG69]. (2017). National Institute for Care and Excellence. London. Retrieved from https://www.nice.org.uk/guidance/ng69

Linna, M. S., Raevuori, A., Haukka, J., Suvisaari, J. M., Suokas, J. T., & Gissler, M. (2014). Pregnancy, obstetric, and perinatal health outcomes in eating disorders. *American Journal of Obstetrics and Gynecology*, *211*(4), 392.e1–392.e8. https://doi.org/10.1016/j.ajog.2014.03.067

Martinez-Olcina, M., Rubio-Arias, J. A., Reche-Garcia, C., Leyva-Vela, B., Hernandez-Garcia, M., Jose Hernandez-Morante, J., & Martinez-Rodriguez, A. (2020). Eating disorders in pregnant and breastfeeding women: A systematic review. *Medicina (Kaunas, Lithuania)*, *56*(7), 352. https://doi.org/10.3390/medicina56070352

National Maternity Review. (2016). Better Births: Improving outcomes of maternity services in England – A five year forward view for maternity care.

Pan, J. R., Li, T. Y., Tucker, D., & Chen, K. Y. (2022). Pregnancy outcomes in women with active anorexia nervosa: A systematic review. *Journal of Eating Disorders*, *10*(25). https://doi.org/10.1186/s40337-022-00551-8

Public Health England. (2018). Making the case for pre-conceptual care. Retrieved from https://www.gov.uk/government/publications/preconception-care-making-the-case

Public Health England. (2019). Health of women before and during pregnancy: Health behaviours, risk factors and inequalities. Retrieved from https://assets.publishing.service.gov.uk/government/uploads/system/uploads/attachment_data/file/844210/Health_of_women_before_and_during_pregnancy_2019.pdf

Scottish Government. (2017). *The Best Start: Five year plan for maternity and neonatal care*. Retrieved from https://www.gov.scot/publications/best-start-five-year-forward-plan-maternity-neonatal-care-scotland/

Stringer, & Furber, C. (2019). Eating disorders in pregnancy: Practical considerations for the midwife. *British Journal of Midwifery*, 27(3), 146–150. https://doi.org/10.12968/bjom.2019.27.3.146

The Nursing and Midwifery Council. (2019). Standards of proficiency for midwives - The Nursing and Midwifery Council. Retrieved from nmc.org.uk

Tuomainen, H., Cross-Bardell, L., Bhoday, M., Qureshi, N., & Kai, J. (2013). Opportunities and challenges for enhancing preconception health in primary care: qualitative study with women from ethnically diverse communities. *British Medical Journal open*, *3*(7), e002977. https://doi.org/10.1136/bmjopen-2013-002977

Index

Note that page numbers in **bold** represent tables and boxes.